THE

EVERYTHING

GUIDE TO
SPICES FOR HEALTH

Dear Reader,

I hope with this book you see your spice rack in a whole new
light and develop a deeper appreciation for spices and their
therapeutic attributes. I want you to discover the beneficial
role spices can have in improving your health, your diet, and
your palate. Spices (and culinary herbs) can have a large
application in your diet, health, and wellness. Some of the
spices you may know, while others might be completely new
to you. I hope you enjoy this book.

Best wishes,

Michelle Robson-Garth

Welcome to the EVERYTHING Series!

These handy, accessible books give you all you need to tackle a difficult project, gain a new hobby, or even brush up on something you learned back in school but have since forgotten. You can choose to read from cover to cover or just pick out information from our four useful boxes.

 Alerts

Urgent warnings

 Facts

Important snippets of information

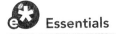 **Essentials**

Quick handy tips

 Questions

Answers to common questions

When you're done reading, you can finally say you know **EVERYTHING®**!

PUBLISHER Karen Cooper

MANAGING EDITOR, EVERYTHING® SERIES Lisa Laing

COPY CHIEF Casey Ebert

ACQUISITIONS EDITOR Eileen Mullan

ASSOCIATE DEVELOPMENT EDITOR Eileen Mullan

EVERYTHING® SERIES COVER DESIGNER Erin Alexander

Visit the entire Everything® series at *www.everything.com*

THE
EVERYTHING
GUIDE TO
SPICES FOR
HEALTH

A complete guide to the natural health-
boosting benefits of everyday spices

Michelle Robson-Garth, BHSc

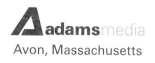

Avon, Massachusetts

An Everything® Series Book.
Everything® and everything.com® are registered trademarks of F+W Media, Inc.

Published by
Adams Media, a division of F+W Media, Inc.
57 Littlefield Street, Avon, MA 02322. U.S.A.
www.adamsmedia.com

ISBN 10: 1-4405-9317-5
ISBN 13: 978-1-4405-9317-8
eISBN 10: 1-4405-9318-3
eISBN 13: 978-1-4405-9318-5

Printed in the United States of America.

10 9 8 7 6 5 4 3 2 1

This book is intended as general information only, and should not be used to diagnose or treat any health condition. In light of the complex, individual, and specific nature of health problems, this book is not intended to replace professional medical advice. The ideas, procedures, and suggestions in this book are intended to supplement, not replace, the advice of a trained medical professional. Consult your physician before adopting any of the suggestions in this book, as well as about any condition that may require diagnosis or medical attention. The author and publisher disclaim any liability arising directly or indirectly from the use of this book.

Many of the designations used by manufacturers and sellers to distinguish their products are claimed as trademarks. Where those designations appear in this book and F+W Media, Inc. was aware of a trademark claim, the designations have been printed with initial capital letters.

Cover images © Ivan Kmit/Anna Kucherova/Eldin Muratovic/Anton Ignatenco/jirkaejc/Ekaterina Fribus/pakhnyushchyy/nito500/George Tsartsianidis/Andrii Gorulko/Marilyn Barbone/Grigory Lukyanov/ Andrii Gorulko/melpomen/Valentyn Volkov/Wim Wyloeck/Anton Ignatenco/photographieundmehr/Sommai Larkjit/123RF.

This book is available at quantity discounts for bulk purchases.
For information, please call 1-800-289-0963.

Dedication

This book is dedicated to my parents and my family, who have always supported and encouraged me in whatever I choose to do.

Acknowledgments

Thank you to the publisher and everyone from Adams Media, including Eileen Mullan, for this opportunity. I would also like to acknowledge the help of Samantha Marks for her inspiration, helpful advice, reviewing, and her quote; Amanda Henham for her quote and assistance; Giselle Demetry and Renee Jones for going over my work tirelessly; and to Clara Bitcon for her quote and inspiration as well.

Sarah Robins for her assistance and help early on; Srijaya Sriharan for teaching me about Malaysian cuisine and for sharing some of her recipes; Geraldine Headley and Lauren Burns for sharing recipes; and Lauren for reviewing, editing, and her quote. Thank you to Helen Padarin for her quote and inspiration over the years.

Thank you to Kelli Benjamin for her quote and all her help. To Susan Marryatt, Rebecca Van Horssen, Jasmine King, and Linda Spirou for reviewing chapters. Thank you to Dr. Becki Milani for helping me with the traditional Chinese medicine information. To Dr. Ram Kishor Deshwal for his assistance with information on Ayurveda. Thank you to Rosemary Gladstar and Dover Publications for allowing me to reference their works. Thank you also to my family, especially my parents and grandparents, for all their help with editing, reading, and reviewing, and for their support.

Contents

The Top 10 Reasons You Should Add Some Spice to Your Life

1. Spices can help make your skin more beautiful and healthier.

2. Spices can aid your digestive system to help break down and absorb your food.

3. Spices may help you get your appetite back if you are experiencing low hunger levels.

4. Spices can help reduce flatulence and bloating.

5. Spices can help improve the general health of your cardiovascular system.

6. Spices are easily found and can be bought at most grocery stores.

7. You can add spices to your diet to expand your palate.

8. Spices can improve metabolic health and weight loss.

9. Spices can help reduce inflammation and pain in the body.

10. Spices can help you prevent and recover from the common cold and flu.

Introduction

When you think of spices, you might think of the spice rack hanging on your kitchen wall, and all the different jars and bottles you've used in your cooking. Spices can do so much more than just flavor your favorite dish. Spices have been used for medicinal purpose for thousands of years. They play an important role in healing and health in many cultures.

Because your health is generally thought to be improved by your diet, or the food you eat, many believe that what you eat can play a role in preventing many modern health complaints and conditions. What you put into your body can impact your body's health. That's why choosing to add different healing spices and herbs to your diet can vastly improve your overall health.

In this book, you will not only discover how to use spices to cook exciting new recipes, but you will also learn the many applications of spices and how they can impact the health of various body systems, and may help relieve symptoms of illness. Interest in natural remedies is increasing and with good reason. According to the National Health Interview Survey released in 2008, 38 percent of U.S. adults over the age of eighteen and about 12 percent of children have used complementary and alternative medicine (CAM). In CAM, herbs and spices are used as a part of the diet for medicinal purposes. Nutritional plants have been a major part of almost every culture in one way or another for years. In fact, herbal medicines were originally a part of medical pharmacopeias. These days, the main forms of complementary medicines used are nutritional and herbal products, as well as massage, acupuncture, naturopathy, and yoga. When used correctly in the right amounts, and when suited to an individual's health, CAM in forms like herbs and spices are very safe and beneficial.

Don't be afraid to experiment with new spices and flavors, but be sure to do your research about every new herb or spice you introduce into your diet.

Spices have many uses to help support good health. From helping to reduce inflammation and pain to supporting digestive health and improving memory, spices can offer tasty additions to your diet as well as benefits that may extend to the whole family. In the next few chapters, you'll explore a variety of herbs and spices, and learn how the right combinations can help you feel your best.

CHAPTER 1

Introduction to the Benefits of Spices

Spices have a variety of healing properties, nutrients, and actions that can be employed in many ways to improve health. The benefits of spices are numerous; they can add flavor, improve digestion, be anti-inflammatory, support the health of your cardiovascular system, and improve your brain health, mood, and immune system. Spices have played a significant role throughout history, not only in the traditional and signature dishes of cultures around the world but in many systems of medicine as well.

What Are Spices?

Although herbs and spices come from medicinal plants, what some define as "herbs" and "spices" may be quite different. Generally speaking, spices are from parts other than the above ground (leafy) parts of edible plants and are usually dried. However, this book includes some culinary herbs that are leaves, as they are commonly used in cooking (sometimes alongside spices) and also have medicinal benefits. These leafy herbs include rosemary leaves, bay leaves, and sage leaves. In this book the word *spices* has been used to describe culinary herbs, as well as what you would commonly call spices.

The Botany of Spices

Knowing what parts of plants are used as spices and getting the correct botanically sourced plant is important, as not all plants are edible and safe. Certain plants are more therapeutic than others. While many herbs and spices may be used in the same ways, and some plants may taste similar, the botany, plant family, and therapeutic and culinary uses of plants can be quite varied. You may be surprised to learn that the identification of true herb and spice parts is not straightforward. For example, some plant parts that we may regard as seeds botanically are actually fruits, such as black pepper.

Herbs and spices botanically speaking come from:

- Arils
- Barks
- Flowers
- Fruits
- Gums
- Resins
- Roots and rhizomes
- Seeds
- Stems

List of Spices

The four major types of herbs and spices that you may already be familiar with are flowers, leaves, seeds, and fruits.

There are many edible and medicinal flowering plants and flowers, some of which are used for flavoring food as well as for medicinal purposes. Some are even used for culinary decoration. Leaves are the aerial parts. "Herbs" usually come from the more herbaceous and green parts of plants.

The seeds are the section of the plant with the most energy and growth potential. They are often a dense source of food for humans and animals alike. We typically think of fruits as being sweet, but that is not always the case. Fruits are usually the nutritious encasing for seeds, which attract animals, birds, and humans to consume them, resulting in the seeds being spread around the earth for germination of plant communities. The following list details the parts of the spice that are used and their botanical names:

FLOWERS
- Calendula (*Calendula officinalis*)
- Clove, a flower bud (*Syzygium aromaticum*)
- Hibiscus (*Hibiscus rosa-sinensis*)
- Rose (*Rosa spp.*)
- Roselle (*Hibiscus sabdariffa*)

LEAVES
- Bay leaf (*Laurus nobilis*)
- Curry leaf (*Murraya koenigii*)
- Kaffir lime leaf (*Citrus hystrix*)
- Rosemary (*Rosmarinus officinalis*)
- Sage (*Salvia officinalis*)
- Thyme (*Thymus vulgaris*)

SEEDS
- Ajowan (*Trachyspermum ammi*)
- Black mustard (*Brassica nigra*)
- Brown mustard (*Brassica juncea*)
- Caraway (*Carum carvi*)
- Cardamom (*Elettaria cardamomum*)
- Cocoa/cacao (*Theobroma cacao*)
- Coriander (*Coriandrum sativum*)
- Cumin (*Cuminum cyminum*)
- Dill seed (*Anethum graveolens*)
- Fennel (*Foeniculum vulgare*)
- Fenugreek (*Trigonella foenum-graecum*)
- Nigella seed (*Nigella sativa*)
- Nutmeg (*Myristica fragrans*)
- Szechuan pepper (*Zanthoxylum simulans*)
- Vanilla (*Vanilla planifolia*)
- Wild celery seed (*Apium graveolens*)
- Yellow mustard (*Brassica alba*)

PODS

- Carob pod (*Ceratonia siliqua*)

BARKS

- Ceylon cinnamon (*Cinnamomum zeylanicum*)
- Chinese cassia cinnamon (*Cinnamomum cassia*)

ROOTS AND RHIZOMES

- Astragalus (*Astragalus membranaceus*)
- Galangal (*Alpinia galanga, Languas galanga, Alpinia officinarum*)
- Ginger (*Zingiber officinale*)
- Horseradish (*Armoracia rusticana*)
- Licorice (*Glycyrrhiza glabra*)
- Turmeric (*Curcuma longa*)

STEMS

- Wasabi (*Eutrema japonicum*)

ARILS

- Mace (*Myristica fragrans*)

STYLES AND STIGMAS

- Saffron (*Crocus sativus*)

FRUITS

- Allspice (*Pimenta dioica*)
- Aniseed (*Pimpinella anisum*)
- Black peppercorns (*Piper nigrum*)
- Cayenne pepper/paprika/chile (*Capsicum annum; Capsicum frutescens; Capsicum spp.* varieties)
- Juniper berries (*Juniperus communis*)
- Star anise (*Illicium verum*)
- Sumac (*Rhus coriaria*)

BULBS/CLOVES
- Garlic (*Allium sativum*)
- Onion (*Allium cepa*)

RESINS (RESINS ARE THE SAP FROM PLANTS)
- Frankincense (*Boswellia serrata*)
- Mastic (*Pistacia lentiscus*)
- Myrrh (*Commiphora myrrha, Commiphora molmol*)

A Brief History of Spices and Medicinal Plants

For thousands of years, plants have been used as food and medicine. Some plants were more successfully used (and safer) than others, and have stood the test of time, whereas others have fallen out of favor, sometimes due to negative, unhealthy effects. Much of the ancient plant matter that was used medicinally is still included in modern and traditional diets, and can be found in many herbalists' dispensaries.

The medicinal values of plants, as well the benefits of nature, have been studied by many early philosophers, doctors, witches, mothers, and natural healers. These important figures include the Greek physician Pedanius Dioscorides (A.D. 40–90), author of *De Materia Medica*; Hippocrates, "the father of medicine" (460–377 B.C.); and Claudius Galen (A.D. 130–200), the Greek philosopher and physician, to name a few. There was also the Iranian philosopher Avicenna (A.D. 980–1037), a medical writer and author of *The Book of Healing*, and the English physician and herbalist Nicholas Culpeper (A.D. 1616–1654). From the East, traditional Chinese medicine and Indian Ayurvedic medicine has made a considerable contribution to the understanding of the healing properties of plant material and the power of nature.

In his *Method of Medicine*, Books 1–4 (2011), Galen notes that spices were used as treatments for illness, sometimes taking the form of "formentations" or poultices, or in extracted oils. He wrote about cumin being suitable "in case[s] of inflations involving the stomach and viscera." He also mentioned cardamom, cinnamon, fenugreek, pepper, coriander, and roses.

Avicenna wrote medically themed books, including those that mentioned herbal medicines, such as *The Canon of Medicine*. He also discussed other topics, such as mathematics, philosophy, and astronomy.

Physician and herbalist Nicholas Culpeper described in his book, now called *Culpeper's Complete Herbal*, a vast *materia medica* of medicinal plants. He wrote about many of the medicinal plants in England, many of which are still regarded as medicinal today, and described such spices as cinnamon, cassia, galangal, cloves, long pepper, ginger, mace, nutmeg, garlic, saffron, and rose, and how they act within body.

Medieval Europe

According to the *Korean Journal of Medical History*, the use of spices in medieval Europe was based on the theories and works of Hippocrates and Galen. During the plague, people were told to boil meat in spices, wine, and vinegar, and spices were used as treatments as well.

 Fact

Some authors assert that in the Middle Ages spices were used to disguise "off" meat, though some authors dispute this claim. Jack Turner, author of the book *Spice: The History of a Temptation*, suggests that spices were used more to disguise the excess use of salt.

How Spice Racks Came About

When looking at spices in your cupboard or on the supermarket shelf, it is hard to imagine the lengths that past explorers had to go to in obtaining these much-prized and sought-after ingredients. The historical significance of how they came to be used and traded is as important as their culinary journey to your plate today, as the spice trade helped shape the modern world. The quest for spices has played a huge part in world history. They originated from all around the world and from diverse cultures.

In modern times herbs and spices are so readily available that it is hard to think of them as foreign currency, but historically they played a big part in trade. Each country has its own unique relationship with various spices, too, depending on how and when they were first procured or produced, and how they were used. The history of spices isn't as one-dimensional as one may think.

Important People in Spice Trade and History

Many people were involved in the "discovery" and history of spices (and riches) in the New World, now called the West Indies. Christopher Columbus from Spain was one of the first players. After many fruitless expeditions, he found the chili plant ("chili pepper") in Central America. He wrongly thought that he had found cinnamon and pepper, as he believed he had arrived in India.

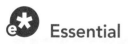 **Essential**

Allspice, another precious spice, is native to America. It was black pepper that had driven many of these explorers on their quest for spices.

The course that Portuguese explorer Vasco da Gama followed in 1497 down the east coast of Africa and on to India was almost completely uncharted. During his voyage, he found numerous spices including black pepper and turmeric. He also discovered cinnamon in Sri Lanka (formerly known as Ceylon). Da Gama brought these spices with him in his travels along the Cape of Good Hope in South Africa, which helped spread spices into Africa.

According to European history, nutmeg and mace were originally discovered in Banda, Indonesia, also known as the Spice Islands by the Dutch. The isolated Banda Islands in Indonesia were the scene of bitter battles, all for the sake of a single spice: nutmeg. Years ago, this group of ten islands were the only source of this rare spice, prompting years of fighting known as the "Nutmeg Wars." The islands were claimed at different times by the Portuguese, the English, and the Dutch.

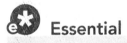 **Essential**

Another spice, cardamom, was found in Malabar, along with certain types of cinnamon, ginger, pepper, and cloves.

At times, the spice trade was very deadly for those who were involved. It spanned centuries and countries including Egypt, India, the Spice Islands (specifically the Moluccas), the Americas, the Middle East, Asia, Holland, Africa, and Spain, and ultimately helped form the world as we know it today.

Flavors of the World

Certain spices and herbs are an integral part of most cultures and cuisines. Global diets are constantly evolving due to the multicultural integration of the world, but there are some flavor combinations that are still very classic and true to certain cultures. In fact, your spice cupboard may have many spices that originated from many continents. While different cultures often use the same spices, most use them in varying ways. Some have their own distinct cuisines, and most national dishes would not be the same without a certain herb or spice. For example, turmeric is the key ingredient in many Indian curries. Nowadays foreign spices are conveniently available to us at grocery stores, spice shops, markets, and online.

India

Spices have long been a part of Indian diets. Their usage varies based on the religions, traditions, and cuisines in specific regions. Certain areas may use more chili than others, for example. Black pepper is native to this country and until the introduction of the chili by the Portuguese traders, it was the main spice used to add heat and pungency to dishes.

Common Indian spices include turmeric, ginger, curry leaves, bay leaves, peppercorns, fenugreek, garlic, ajowan, urad dahl, asafetida, cumin, coriander, and chili. Typical mixes of spices used in cooking include garam masala (which means "hot spice"), masala chai ("spicy tea"), and panch phoron ("five spices").

China

Chinese cooking makes use of many spices. Garlic, cinnamon, star anise, ginger, cloves, chili, licorice, and Szechuan pepper are used in traditional Chinese meals. Many spices are also used in traditional Chinese medicine.

Thailand and Malaysia

Typical ingredients used in Thai cooking include coconut milk, kaffir lime leaves, lime, ginger, garlic, lemongrass, chili, and galangal root, as well as fresh herbs such as coriander, Thai mint, and Thai basil.

Malaysian dishes use an amalgamation of flavors from cuisines such as India and China, as well as Nyonya, which is a blend of Chinese and Malaysian ethnic flavors. Ingredients used include tamarind, black pepper, ginger, garlic, star anise, galangal, coconut, cassia cinnamon, cardamom, and chili.

Indonesia and Korea

Indonesia is home to nutmeg, mace, and cloves. Traditional Indonesian cuisine typically uses sweet and sour flavors and includes staple starches such as rice, among other grains and ingredients such as soy, beans and bean products, coconut milk products, nuts, seeds, fish, and fresh fruits and vegetables. Indonesian cooking is also known to use coriander, and spices such as cumin, ginger, garlic, and chili. Chili and garlic are important ingredients in kimchi, the much-loved spicy Korean dish made with fermented cabbage.

America and Mediterranean Countries

Some of the medicinal plants that are used as spices today were used medicinally in certain Native American cultures. According to Daniel E. Moerman, author of *Native American Ethnobotany*, these plants include roses, sage, juniper, black pepper, cayenne, and chili pepper, which were used by a number of tribes for different purposes. Vanilla pod and bell pepper (capsicum) are native to America. Chili, and its many varieties, and cocoa come from Mexico.

The "Mediterranean diet" includes foods that are rich in polyunsaturated fatty acids such as olives and olive oil, along with seafood, grains and legumes, nuts and seeds, and plenty of fruits and vegetables. This, of course, differs between countries and traditional foods used.

The Middle East, North Africa, and Africa

The Middle East and North Africa includes countries such as Morocco, Egypt, Tunisia, Iran (Persia), Pakistan, Iraq, Israel, Kuwait, and Lebanon. The different spices and flavors used in these areas include cinnamon, rose, sumac, licorice, black pepper, coriander, cumin, cardamom, and saffron. Fresh herbs such as peppermint are used as well.

African countries use a range of spices including chili, cinnamon, barberry, pepper, coriander seed, berbere (an Ethiopian spice blend), paprika, fennel, ginger, rose petals, cloves, mustard, cardamom, turmeric, and cumin.

Australia

Very few native Australian spices and herbs are used in everyday Australian cooking. This is because many Australians use spices from other countries. In addition, the population of Australia is very multicultural. However, native spices and herbs are gaining popularity. A few of the more unique Australian foods and spices include lemon myrtle leaves (*Backhousia citriodora*), wattleseed (*Acacia aneura*), native pepper (*Tasmannia lanceolata*), bush tomato (*Solanum centrale*), finger lime (*Citrus australasica*), eucalyptus leaves (*Eucalyptus globulus*), and macadamia nuts (*Macadamia integrifolia*).

Systems of Traditional Medicine

Systems of traditional medicine are still used as an initial response to help heal ailments, as well as to maintain and to support health. According to the World Health Organization (WHO), "countries in Africa, Asia, and Latin America use traditional medicine (TM) to help meet some of their primary healthcare needs. In Africa, up to 80 percent of the population uses traditional medicine for primary healthcare. In industrialized countries, traditional, herbal, and nutritional medicines are termed Complementary and Alternative Medicine (CAM)."

An Introduction to Traditional Systems of Natural Medicine

Almost every country has its own customary, healing medicine systems based on nature. Plants, and sometimes animal products, are often used to manage health issues in various ways, especially in indigenous cultures. Thousands of plants have medicinal and nutritional properties and can be used therapeutically, though some plants are more popular in certain systems than others. Of course, plants are also used as foods and are medicinal and nutritious just by being part of the diet.

Western Herbal Medicine

Western herbal medicine (WHM) uses a combination of long-established, current, and up-to-date evidence-based information as it becomes available on herbal medicine. Western herbal medicine follows information from past herbalists as well as finding new applications and uses. It also aims to provide cautionary information for herbal medicines based on scientific literature that is available.

Herbal medicine is the science and art of using plants and herbal medicines to improve health and well-being. WHM takes into account the health of the individual including any medical conditions, lifestyle, stress, diet, and any medications that could potentially interact with the herbal remedies prescribed. Once this is established, practitioners may recommend herbs that may improve their condition.

Naturopathy

Naturopathy is a system that combines the use of herbal medicine, dietary therapies, nutritional medicine, massage, and lifestyle adjustments. It aims to view and treat the body as a whole.

Naturopathy is used in many countries including the United States, Australia, Canada, the United Kingdom, and India. It can vary across these countries depending on laws and what is included in each country's *materia medica* (herbal information), traditional practices, and the scientific data and literature available to them.

Naturopaths abide by the following tenants, originally derived from Hippocrates. These include:

- *Primum non nocere*: First do no harm.
- *Vis medicatrix naturae*: The healing power of nature.
- *Tolle causam*: To identify and treat the cause.
- *Docere*: Doctor as teacher.
- *Tolle totum*: Treat the whole person and individually.
- Prevention of illness, wherever possible.

Ayurveda

Next to allopathic medicine, Ayurveda is the main traditional medicine system in India. The word *Ayurveda* can be translated to mean "the Science of Life." Ayurveda combines the use of herbal medicine, yoga, and dietary therapies. Ayurveda acknowledges three constitutional states, called doshas. These states are vata, pitta, and kapha. Ayurveda also uses the five elements: earth, ether, fire, water, and wind. In Ayurvedic medicine, you are assigned a constitution based on which one matches your individualized pattern of health. This then determines what foods, herbs, dietary therapies, or other treatments may be suitable for you.

Traditional Chinese Medicine (TCM)

Traditional Chinese medicine includes therapies such as acupuncture (including cupping, moxibustion, and Qi Gong, which is similar to tai chi), herbal medicine, dietary therapies, lifestyle therapies, and a type of massage called tui na. There is some crossover between medicinal plants used in China and India. Elements of the earth and the energetics of plants (if a food or herb is warming or cooling) are also considered in TCM. Some of the spices used therapeutically in TCM cooking, and in herbal medicines, include rose petals, which can be made into tisanes; black sesame seeds, which can be added to soups and stews; goji berry (or wolf-berry); and chrysanthemum. According to Becki Milani, doctor of Chinese medicine, some of the spices used in TCM, and their corresponding Pinyin names, include fresh ginger (*sheng jiang*), licorice (*gan cao*), cinnamon bark (*rou gui*), black pepper (*hu jiao*), chili (*gan jiang*), and peppermint (*bo he*). She also explains that in TCM, herbs and spices would be prescribed to a patient based on an underlying TCM pattern, which may be determined based on investigations and physical signs such as pulse.

Middle Eastern Traditional Medicine

In an article in *Evidence-Based Complementary and Alternative Medicine* in 2006, Hassan Azaizeh and Bashar Saad detail some of the herbal medicines used in the eastern region of the Mediterranean. Almost 300 plants are used for medicinal purposes. The herbal medicines mentioned that have been used as food and sometimes as teas as well as medicine include *Nigella sativa* (nigella seed), *Olea europaea* (olive leaf), *Teucrium polium* (felty germander), *Pimpinella anisum* (aniseed), *Trigonella foenum-graecum* (fenugreek), and *Silybum marianum* (milk thistle).

Healing Properties of Spices

Spices sometimes seem like the unsung heroes, relegated to the back of your cupboard, while herbs reap all the glory, both in their dried form or in the crisper in the fridge. Spices, however, are very medicinal, nutritious, and delicious. They should be a celebrated part of your diet for the way they add flavor as well as for their potential therapeutic qualities.

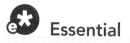 **Essential**

The makeup of medicinal and nutritious plants and their chemicals heal and help humans in a variety of ways and are used in many traditional healing systems. Plants are able to heal through their constituents, nutrients, and actions. These constituents and nutrients can affect the body in hundreds if not thousands of ways. The herbal actions are a result of the chemical substances and physical attributes of the plants.

Food As Medicine

Food, herbs, and spices can have powerful medicinal properties. "Food as Medicine" is the concept of using a nutritious diet or modifying it in such a way as to make it possible to support and aid the body within certain illnesses or health complaints. It also may help to prevent certain health conditions, where possible. Some believe eating "whole foods" can help achieve this goal. Whole foods are unprocessed, unrefined foods that are nutrient-rich. They include fresh meats, eggs, full-fat dairy products, nuts and seeds, fresh fruits, vegetables, and whole grains. They are nutritious, minimally processed, and unrefined.

Actions of Spices

Spices (and herbs) can be categorized according to certain "actions" and properties. These are based on how medicinal plants react in the body and are sourced from a number of *materia medica*, along with anecdotal, empirical, and scientific evidence.

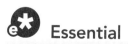 **Essential**

Materia medica means "medical material." *Materia medica* are often developed from historical documents, including the works of Nicholas Culpeper and other herbalists.

Actions of therapeutic plants include analgesic, antibacterial, antiemetic, anti-inflammatory, antimicrobial, antioxidant, antispasmodic, antiviral, astringent, adaptogen, adrenal tonic, bitter, carminative, demulcent, emollient, expectorant, hepatoprotective, hypotensive, immune modulating, mucolytic, nervine, nootropic, and spasmolytic. New actions of medicinal plants are continuing to be discovered through ongoing studies.

Constituents in Spices

You may know certain spices for their tastes or aromas, but this is only one aspect of what they offer to a meal. Different plants contain constituents, all of which can have different actions, even among plants within the same family. In fact, for some plants, not all constituents have been discovered and isolated. Practitioners and spice consumers can look to information from traditional and modern herbal medicine texts to find out more about the benefits.

Types of Constituents

Volatile (essential) oils and oleoresins are some of the constituents in spices that contribute to their characteristic and delicious aromas and tastes. Essential oils are often extracted and concentrated to be used in aromatherapy for topical use, for example diluted in massage oil, or to be used in oil burners to release their essential oils in the air for therapeutic inhalation. Other constituents in spices include alkaloids (e.g., piperine in black pepper), sesquiterpene ketones (such as turmerones in turmeric), polysaccharides (such as in cinnamon), tannins (found in black and green tea), antioxidants such as flavonoids and polyphenols, coumarins, saponins, and xanthines. This is only a small list; medicinal plants contain many more constituents than this book can cover.

Synergy and Complexity of Whole Spices

While herbs and spices are wonderful on their own, they can work very well together in food and with one another, creating a greater synergistic and healing effect. While pharmaceutical drugs may have limited ingredients, spices (and herbs) are extremely complex and contain thousands of constituents; not all of them have been named or their properties identified. These constituents sometimes help form a plant's delicious aroma, taste, and therapeutic benefits. Medicinal plants can also have a synergistic and even more therapeutic effect when used in with other complimentary plants.

Nutrients in Spices

Spices are often thought of as nourishing as they come from storage parts of plants such as roots and seeds. Some spices are rich in phytonutrients (plant nutrients) such as flavonoids, as well as other nutrients you may be familiar with including vitamin C, which is in chili, rose hip, and goji berries; magnesium from cocoa, coffee, and black sesame seed; as well as vitamins A and E; calcium; and the minerals iron and zinc, which have been found in black pepper.

Throughout this book you will learn about how spices may be applied to reduce inflammation, how you can enhance your immune system with them, and how they may help improve gut function, brain, joint, and skin health; aid weight loss; how they may help improve the overall health of cardiovascular system; and may be suitable to help support certain chronic diseases.

Spiritual Aspects of Spices

Spices are mentioned in many spiritual texts. For many, spirituality is a big part of life and culture. Spirituality and piety is thought to have a positive effect on well-being and health. It may also be a part of how some people cope with life.

Religious Uses of Spices

Many religious and spiritual works mention spices and herbs, including the Bible, the Torah, and the Koran. There are also other religions and faiths that mention herbs and spices.

The Torah and Old Testament of the Bible

There are references to many spices in the Torah, which includes the following books in the Old Testament: Genesis, Exodus, Leviticus, Numbers, and Deuteronomy. You may associate some spices with Christian holidays such as Christmas or other celebratory days. The Bible talks about many spices including, and most famously, frankincense and myrrh, and also the natural mineral gold, which are said to have been given to Jesus upon his birth by the three wise men. Other spices mentioned include cinnamon, saffron, the balm of Gilead, wormwood, cumin, dill, cassia, coriander, and salt. According to the Bible, upon Jesus' death, his body was wrapped in linen along with certain (unnamed) spices. Spices were used as perfumes and many had spiritual meanings.

Specific Spices Mentioned in the Bible

Myrrh is often mentioned in the Bible. In Proverbs 7:17, myrrh, along with aloe and cinnamon, are referred to as perfumes. Myrrh is also mentioned in the books Song of Solomon, Mark, Psalms, John, Genesis, Exodus, and Ester.

Balm of Gilead, also known as balsam, is referred to in the Bible as well. It is mentioned in Genesis and twice in the book of Jeremiah. In the Bible it says that the Queen of Sheba gave balsam (*Commiphora gileadensis*) to King Solomon as a gift. It was grown in Israel and has been used as a perfume in the past, though it is not often used these days.

Frankincense (*Boswellia serrata*) is mentioned in many books of the Bible, including Leviticus, Song of Solomon, and Nehemiah, as an important spice and perfume. It is also used today as an essential oil and in herbal medicine preparations.

 Fact

Catholic priests swing around thuribles within the church, which burn incense. Different churches use different incenses in their thuribles.

Spiritual Paths, Traditional Cultures, and the Use of Spices

Spices can also be a part of nonreligious spiritual paths and traditional cultures, which may have a spiritual aspect to them.

Witchcraft

Witches are thought to have used herbal medicines for various healing ways as well. Some forms of witchcraft such as hedgewitchery use spices in ritualistic and intuitive ways. They may be chosen based on a seasonal calendar called the Wheel of the Year. Spices have specific meanings and can be used differently throughout this calendar, and the Gregorian calendar year as well. According to one practitioner of hedgewitchery, Alison Bramich, spices may be used in food, in potions, ground into incense, smoked on coals, or macerated in water or alcohol to make a room spray or even to be used as a wash for the body or the feet.

Some of the spices used in witchcraft are considered to have temperaments and they may be associated with the sun due to their warming nature. Other spices (and foods) may be associated with the four elements: earth, fire, water, and air. Examples are saffron and calendula (which are both associated with the sun), myrrh, frankincense, galangal, and dragon's blood, the latter containing a bright red, sweet-smelling resin, which is linked to the element of fire.

These are just a few. Practitioners of witchcraft use spices that are believed to increase clairsentience, that is, clarity of life, and to help improve their understanding of their own body. Spices have many applications in witchcraft. Those that are derived from roots, such as licorice, and barks, such as cinnamon, are often considered to be "grounding" and are thought to help increase the body's energy from the root chakra.

Traditional Western Herbal Medicine

Nicholas Culpeper's writings also had a spiritual aspect, particularly in the descriptions of herbs. Culpeper used astrology to describe connections between herbal medicines and how they may suit how the body functions, as well as how they benefit and influence the body.

White sage (*Salvia apiana*) is often thought to have spiritual properties. It is used ritualistically as an ingredient in smudge sticks. White sage is believed to have an emotional and energy-cleansing action to it, and some believe it is thought to release negative energy and bad spirits. White sage is used in combination with other herbs in smudge sticks.

Herbal medicines and nutritious plants have a long tradition throughout various cultures, religions, and spiritual practices. They are still being used today for the advantage of human (and even animal) health. Let's celebrate the wonder of nature and continue this exploration of how you can make spices a part of your diet and healthy lifestyle.

CHAPTER 2

Cooking with Spices

Spices can be added to your diet for their health-promoting benefits. Not only can they be used in food but they can also be used topically in certain preparations. Spices can be cooked into a meal to flavor it. They can be used in aromatherapy as essential oils (which have had certain constituents called volatile oils extracted), infused into oils for cooking or for use on the body, depending on the spice, or prepared as infusions (teas) or as decoctions. Spices can also be made into marinades for meat or rubs to flavor roast vegetables or meat. They can be added to syrups to flavor food or to be used as medicinal aids, such as in syrups for coughs. Spices can even be used to make certain beauty treatments. There are endless ways you may make your life a little bit more spicy.

Buying, Storage, and Safety

Spices can easily be found in many grocery stores, as well as at farmers' markets and at certain websites, and of course at spice shops. This depends on what kind of spice you are looking for. Some spices can be more difficult to get your hands on, especially if they are coming from another continent or if they are rare.

Spice Safety

When used in dietary amounts, spices are very safe to consume. It is important to know the correct botanical name of the plant you are buying as some plants may seem similar but have different actions and uses. Buying from reputable sources that sell well-sourced spices is important to ensure you know the origin of the spices, as well as the quality. This also helps to prevent you from buying adulterated spices that have been mixed with undesirable substances, or plant or spice substitutes.

Organic, Sustainable, and Fair-Trade Farming

When buying spices, it is important to be aware of not only where the spices have come from, but also how they have been produced—that is, whether they are organic, biodynamic, sustainably produced, and how they are farmed.

Organic spices are plants that are grown without any kind of pesticide and are free of genetically modified organisms (GMOs). Biodynamic farming is organic farming, which aims to work with the local ecosystem of the land where a plant is farmed and enhances the health of the land and the plants grown on it by a variety of methods. Fair-trade farming takes into account the welfare and the rights of the workers who work on the farms. Sustainable farming takes into account how susceptible certain plants are to extinction and aims to support the growth and sustainability of ecological farming practices.

How Many Spices You Should Buy

It can be a good idea to buy smaller rather than larger quantities of spices. This helps to ensure they stay fresh, especially if you don't think you will use them regularly. Keeping a small amount means they won't lose their flavor or color as readily than if you had a larger amount, which could easily become wasted. This is even more beneficial if you don't feel you will use a certain spice often. It is generally cheaper, too. Certain packets of spices can even be as low as a few dollars. However, you can also buy spices in bulk and share with friends or family, which would make it much more economical.

Is This Spice Fresh?

Like any food, spices need to be kept well to stay fresh. They are best bought in whole forms, for example whole gingerroot, whole nutmeg, and whole cumin seed. Buying whole spices will mean their constituents and nutrients will stay intact longer, and they will taste better, as their surface area has had less exposure to light, heat, and air, which can rapidly deteriorate their nutrients, aromas, and flavors. Simple steps to assess the freshness of the spice include:

- Look at the color. Certain spices are quite vibrant. If their color has become dulled, they may not be as fresh as they once were.
- Smell the spice. They should be fragrant and aromatic. However, if whole, it may be a little bit harder to detect any aroma.
- Taste the spice. If possible, see if you can have a sample of the spice to taste it and see how fresh it is.

How to Store Dried Spices

Spices can be stored in a round metal tin with a lid that contains smaller round metal containers. These are often used in Indian kitchens and are called masala dabba. You can also store dried spices in brown paper bags tied with elastic bands, glass bottles, or even ziplock bags.

Dried spices are best stored in lidded glass containers in a cupboard, to prevent contamination. It is even better if the containers are dark blue or amber colored. This helps to avoid contact with light and anything that could harm the spices. If your container isn't dark, you could try wrapping tin foil around the glass jar to shield the contents from light and sunshine. It is best to avoid storing dried spices in the fridge or freezer to avoid contact with moisture. Moisture may cause the spice to deteriorate. An exception are those that have been made into a cooked paste. If this is the case, then they will stay fresh in the refrigerator for some time.

Storing Fresh Spices

Fresh spices can be wrapped up and stored in airtight containers kept in the refrigerator. This is to prevent them from drying out and developing mold. This is good for fresh spices such as curry leaves, fresh ginger rhizome, fresh turmeric, galangal, and peeled garlic. These can also be cut up into small pieces and frozen in a ziplock bag for later use. You could try freezing fresh spices to be used as a part of a delicious sauce or marinade later.

Preparing Spices and Useful Equipment

You don't need a lot of equipment to add spices to your cooking. In fact, you can get away with very few extra utensils. You may simply need only a glass jar to store them in. A few useful appliances and pieces of equipment include:

- **A sharp knife:** To chop fresh spices such as ginger, turmeric, garlic, horseradish, and onion. Garlic can be smashed with the flat side of a knife and a bit of salt, which aids the physical breakdown of garlic. This is useful when you need to cook a lot of garlic or you find garlic hard to crush.
- **A blender:** To make sauces, marinades, and pastes or powdered spice mixes.
- **A mortar and pestle:** This will allow you to crush or bruise a small amount of spices in an efficient way.
- **A pepper grinder:** Pepper is so much more flavorful and fresh-tasting when ground from whole peppercorns. You can add whole black peppercorns to a grinder to grind and then sprinkle over your meals.
- **A box grater:** This can be used to grate garlic, ginger, turmeric, and other spices derived from roots.

Preparing Herbs and Spices

Herbs and spices can be prepared in a number of ways to enhance their flavor and release their nutritional benefits. Preparations include:

- **Dry roasting:** Some whole spices can be dry roasted in a pan before adding them to meals when cooking, to help release their aromatic essential oils and flavors. They can also be crushed after they are roasted and then added to the base of a meal.

- **Crushing:** Spices can be crushed, for example in a mortar and pestle, in order to break down the cell walls and release the flavors.

- **Grinding:** Spices can be ground, again using a mortar and pestle, or they can be ground in a food processor or blender to make them into a fine powder.

- **Chopping:** Garlic, onion, horseradish, turmeric, and garlic can all be chopped for different meals.

- **Grating:** Fresh spices such as ginger, horseradish, turmeric, and garlic can be grated and mixed into marinades or cooked as a part of a variety of dishes.

- **Infusions and decoctions:** Infusions are a preparation that involves pouring boiled (or room temperature water for delicate herbs) water over a certain herb or spice. Spices can be infused into water as herbal teas. Decoctions are boiled preparations using medicinal plants.

- **Infused oil:** Spices can also be infused into oil. Suitable spices that can be infused include dried ginger, dried garlic, dried chili, and dried turmeric.

- **Infused vinegar:** Spices such as rosemary, thyme, and dried garlic pair well to make an infused vinegar.

- **Infused alcohol:** Spices such as vanilla or cinnamon can be used to flavor alcohol.

- **Infused salt or sugar:** Vanilla beans or cinnamon sticks can be infused in sugar for sweet dishes. Spices such as rosemary or even seaweed can be mixed with salt for flavoring savory dishes.
- **Dried:** Spices can be dried if bought fresh to use later on.

Note: There can be a risk of botulism spores if using fresh spices in an infused oil.

Cooking with Spices

Spices can be prepared in a number of ways to enhance your meals and your health. They are generally cooked but can also be added to different preparations such as soups, stews, curries, teas, breads, sauces, smoothies, and more! The only limitations are your taste buds and your imagination.

You don't need a lot of spices to add variety to your meals. Even a single spice can be used for multiple cuisines and tastes. If you've never used herbs and spices in your cooking, now is the perfect time to start!

Using Spices to Make Tea

The tea plant, *Camellia sinensis*, is used to make black tea and also green tea (the different varieties of green and black tea are just prepared in various ways). You can add spices to black tea for a change in flavor, or you can make herbal infusions with the herbs as the only ingredient. You can also gently simmer the spices (especially woodier parts) for a stronger herbal tea, as these parts need a stronger extraction force. Infusions (tisanes) are usually made with gentler plant parts including petals, flowers, and leaves.

Many common spices can be added to tea or tea mixes including ginger (fresh and dried), fennel seed, star anise, pepper, rose, vanilla, dried orange peel, turmeric, and cardamom, as well as peppermint, sage, and thyme, which are culinary herbs. Chai is another example of a spiced tea.

Spices You Can Use in Curries, Soups, and Stews

Spices are famous for being a key part of curries. The different spices used in soups and curries include chili, star anise, garlic, black pepper, fennel seed, mustard seed, Szechuan peppercorn, cumin, coriander (seed, powder, and the fresh herb), and turmeric.

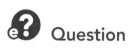 **Alert**

Be careful when adding chili to a soup as the flavor and heat will spread right through the whole dish.

Laksa is a Malaysian soup recipe that includes spices such as garlic, ginger, galangal, chili, onions, and turmeric. Other ingredients include seafood, coconut milk, and noodles. Another popular spice dish is chili con carne, which is a slow-cooked minced meat stew that usually contains spices such as cumin and is also flavored with tomatoes, and sometimes beans.

Question

What kinds of sauces can I make with different spices?
Certain sauces would not be the same without the spices that enhance them. For example, black pepper is used in gravy and traditionally in carbonara sauce, nutmeg is often used in white sauces, and turmeric is used in curry pastes.

Spices You Can Use to Cook with Grains and Meats

Saffron is often used to flavor and color rice. It is sometimes substituted by turmeric to bring a similar bright yellow effect. Calendula flower petals can be used to flavor cooking water when boiling rice as a cheaper alternative to saffron. When cooking meats such as lamb, beef, bison, fowl, and fish, you can use nutmeg, chili, black pepper, cinnamon, cumin, coriander, onion, garlic, and paprika. Spices can be used to enhance and add flavor to meat in conjunction with any cooking method. They can also be used in marinades, dry rubs, and wet rubs.

Spices You Can Use When Making Sweets

There are many different spices you can use when baking. Breads and cakes can be great vehicles for trying new spice combinations. For example, apple strudel uses nutmeg and shortbread uses vanilla. Some traditional spices used in baked goods include cinnamon, cloves, pepper, nutmeg, ginger, vanilla, allspice, saffron, rose, green tea, cocoa, marigold, and cardamom.

Spice Mixes

Many spices can complement others and can be mixed together to create even greater flavor profiles. Don't be afraid to experiment and make your own spice mixes for your favorite meals. Here are a list of popular spice mixes to get started:

- **Cajun chicken spice mix:** Cajun food is hot and spicy and has origins in Southern American cooking. To flavor chicken and other meat, a combination of spices such as garlic, thyme, paprika, white pepper, and cayenne pepper can be mixed together along with celery seed, onion, and bell peppers (capsicum). You can use this in mincemeat or as a dry or wet rub on meat.

- **Jerk spice powder:** A "jerk" spice mix, thought to have originated in Jamaica, is a spicy dry rub or marinade for chicken and other meats such as beef, pork, and seafood that combines a mixture of nutmeg, green onions (or scallions), ginger, allspice, chili, cinnamon, thyme, cloves, sugar, salt, and pepper. After the meat has marinated it is usually barbecued.
- **Baharat spice mix:** Baharat is a Middle Eastern spice mix consisting of cumin seed, paprika, black peppercorns, cloves, nutmeg, cinnamon, and cardamom.
- **Masala chai:** *Masala chai* means "spiced tea." It is a fragrant and aromatic mixture of spices and a particular kind of Indian chai. It includes black tea, green cardamom, fennel, cinnamon, cloves, and ginger. You can also add other spices and flavors such as black peppercorns, star anise, bay leaves, coriander seed, even orange zest or chocolate.
- **Chinese five-spice powder:** Chinese five-spice powder is a mix that includes cloves, cinnamon, star anise, fennel, and pepper.
- **Classic Indian curry powder:** A classic mixture of spices you can use to make an Indian-style curry powder includes turmeric powder, cumin seed, coriander seed, fennel seed, and mustard seed. They can be fried in a pan with a bit of oil before adding meat or vegetables to be cooked.
- **Dukka:** Dukka is a nut, seed, and spice mix that originated in Egypt. Dukka can contain the spice mix baharat or other spices such as cumin seed, coriander seed, fennel seed, and pepper. Nuts and seeds such as sesame seed, almonds, or pistachio nuts may be used. Dukka can be served with olive oil as a dip for bread to pick up the spices.

- **Garam masala:** Garam masala, a North Indian spice mix, is generally only used at the end of curries. It usually contains a mixture of spices including cardamom, coriander, cumin, cinnamon, cloves, and black pepper.
- **Panch phoron:** Panch phoron is an Indian spice mix that contains fenugreek, nigella seed, cumin seed, mustard seed, and fennel seed. You can make this by mixing equal parts together.
- **Ras el hanout:** *Ras el hanout* means "head of the shop" and it is a North African spice blend. It generally contains spices such as ginger, nutmeg, coriander, allspice, cumin, turmeric, paprika, cardamom, cloves, cinnamon, black peppercorns, and cayenne pepper or even saffron.
- **Mulled wine:** Mulled wine can be made by gently steeping red or white wine with spices such as cinnamon, aniseed, cloves, vanilla, or allspice along with fresh fruit such as oranges (or just orange zest), raisins, apples, or berries. Sometimes rose petals are used too.
- **Harissa paste:** Harissa paste is a combination of chilies, roasted capsicum, onion, garlic, vinegar, and oil. It can be used as a condiment or to marinate meat or tofu before roasting or frying.

CHAPTER 3

Spices for a Healthy Immune System

Your immune system is your body's main system of protection against foreign invaders such as bacteria and viruses. It uses a range of chemical processes, as well as physical barriers of the body, that offer you protection and resilience. Your immune system is made up of two parts, innate immunity and adaptive immunity. Sometimes, though, your immune system may need a little help. You can help strengthen your immune system naturally by adjusting your diet and lifestyle. This may be achieved by adding certain foods, herbs, and spices to your daily routine, as well as improving sleep habits and exercise.

Innate Immunity

Your natural, innate immune system is a part of your first line of defense against foreign bodies such as bacteria, toxins, and viruses. This is the part of your immune system you are born with. It includes physical barriers such as the skin, mucous membranes, and processes such as inflammation. The innate immune system is nonspecific. It doesn't care what it fights against; it just works and fights for you without question, against any pathogen, unless your immunity is compromised.

Skin and Mucous Membranes

As mentioned, your body has a number of protective barriers such as the skin and mucous membranes to protect you from pathogens (microorganisms, such as bacteria and fungi), as well as from toxic substances. Your skin, as your outside protective covering, is one of the first barriers of protection you have against outside forces and microbes. Your mucous membranes are another physical barrier that protects you. The mucous membranes line your mouth, nose, throat, gut, internal sex organs, and linings of the respiratory tract. The membranes produce mucus, which is protective, and physically assist with actual collection and removal of dead cells and bacteria. The body removes some of this mucus through mechanisms such as sneezing and coughing.

The Gut, Epithelial Cells, and Bacteria

Your digestive acids also play a role in the immune system by breaking down proteins from food, as well as by breaking down proteins from microbes in the gastrointestinal tract. Cells and bacteria in your gut offer protection as well. Other chemicals that destroy or affect bacteria include your tears and sweat. Your body produces specialized chemicals from epithelial cells that can destroy bacteria, viruses, and fungi.

Inflammation, Phagocytes, and White Blood Cells

Your innate immune system also protects you with cells and processes including inflammation, histamine reactions, cytokines, the complement system, white blood cells, and various kinds of proteins. Phagocytes, which are involved in the process of phagocytosis, are important for the immune system too. Phagocytes can be thought of as the "Pac-Men" of your immune system. They protect you by engulfing pathogens, such as microbes, and destroying them. The Greek meaning of phagocytosis is "to devour." The phagocytes "eat" pathogens to protect your body. They can recognize pathogens by receptors present on their surfaces. The main types of phagocytes are neutrophils, macrophages (which are "Pac-Men"), and monocytes. White blood cells include eosinophils, which protect your body against parasites, basophils, which are activated in times of asthma and allergies due to the histamine reaction, and natural killer cells, which destroy cells that have become infected.

Adaptive Immunity

Adaptive immunity, or the acquired immune system, is developed over time and life by learning and adapting to pathogens. It offers a stronger source of immunity once it develops than the innate immune system.

 Fact

Vaccinations help stimulate this part of your immune system by helping the system to adapt and strengthen itself.

B and T Cells

The adaptive immunity protects you from antigens and learns lessons about these antigens along the way to make your immune system stronger. An antigen is anything that your body recognizes as foreign, such as environmental substances, and microbes such as viruses, bacteria, parasites, or fungi. Antigens are what stimulate your immune system to produce antibodies. Antibodies, or immunoglobulins as they are known, and types of white blood cells called lymphocytes protect your body against these antigens. The adaptive immune system works against specific antigens and it is also able to develop memory against these antigens, so your immune system becomes stronger and more efficient.

Two specialized forms of lymphocytes are the B and T cells. You are born with both these cells. The B and T cells mature in the bone marrow and thymus, respectively. B cells are stimulated by antigens to produce antibodies. There are many kinds of T cells that have specific functions that support your immune system and support the B cells in their work too. Some T cells kill infected cells, others help the immune system, and still other cells help regulate the immune system. These two parts, along with other cells and organs of the body, make up your immune system.

All these cells and systems work together to keep your body healthy by protecting it from invading pathogens, foreign materials, and chemicals.

Foods and Tips for a Healthier Immune System

There are certain lifestyles and dietary elements you can embrace to generally improve the overall robustness and health of your immune system. The immune system needs a number of things to be healthy in addition to a nutritious diet, such as adequate sleep, sunshine, exercise, and stress reduction.

A Nutritious Diet

What you eat, whether good or bad, may affect the health of your immune system. Some foods may have a positive role in immune system health due to their nutrients and phytochemical content. Foods that are generally good for the immune system include adequate intake of animal proteins and products such as red meat, eggs, dairy products, fish, pork, and poultry, due to their abundance of protein and amino acids, zinc, B vitamins, and fat-soluble vitamins.

Other foods that are particularly good for the immune system include fruits and vegetables, especially green leafy and colorful vegetables and a rainbow of brightly colored fruits, fresh nuts and seeds, and various kinds of edible mushrooms and seaweeds. There are also components of the diet that when they are in excess (or deficient) could affect the health of the immune system. For example, excess refined sugar and a deficiency of protein have the potential to affect immune system health.

A Good Night's Sleep

Getting enough sleep is important for many aspects of your health, including your hormonal health and that of your immune system. Melatonin is produced in darkness by the pineal gland while you sleep. Melatonin is a hormone and an antioxidant, meaning it is protective to your cells, and it may be important for reducing oxidative stress in the body. Your body also detoxifies while resting and sleeping, so quality sleep is important for a healthy immune system.

Sunlight

Sunlight is actually protective for your body, to a certain extent, as it enables your body to produce vitamin D. Your body produces vitamin D in your skin, from the stimulation of ultraviolet (UV) light from sunshine. As a hormone, vitamin D, which is technically called calcitriol or 1,25-dihydroxyvitamin D, has many actions and roles in your body, many of which are protective and important for the health of your immune system. Vitamin D is important in growth and development due to its role in maintaining calcium levels and metabolism, skeletal health, and growth.

Vitamin D is thought to have some role in modulating your immune system and possibly antiproliferative effects. Martin Hewison, in *Proceedings of the Nutrition Society* in 2012, says that "immunomodulatory actions of vitamin D have been recognized for over a quarter of a century, but it is only in the last few years that the significance of this to normal human physiology has become apparent." As part of the immune system function, vitamin D influences antimicrobial mechanisms in the body, and T-lymphocyte cell function. You can get small amounts of vitamin D, as a fat-soluble vitamin, from foods such as fatty fish, liver, cod liver oil, and even mushrooms. If exposed under UV light, mushrooms have been shown to produce vitamin D.

Managing Stress

Stress places a great deal of pressure on your immune system and your health. You can think of stress as a "toxin" to the body. In too great an amount it can be detrimental to many systems in your body. Stress can have a systemic unhealthful effect on your whole body, including negative effects on the immune system, your gastrointestinal and endocrine systems, and reproductive system.

A Healthy Body Weight and Exercise

A healthy body weight can have a positive effect on your immune system. This is because fat cells have the potential to produce inflammatory chemicals. A healthy body weight also reduces your chances of many chronic diseases. The hormone leptin modulates energy metabolism and body weight and can affect the immune system. Exercise helps you maintain a healthy body weight. Exercise is anti-inflammatory, helps break down inflammatory chemicals, and helps the body produce endorphins. Exercise is also thought to be beneficial for many health conditions including depression, obesity, and certain joint conditions such as arthritis.

Actions for the Immune System

Herbs and spices can have medicinal effects on your immune system, helping your body to rid itself of foreign invaders. The following list explains what kind of actions medicinal plants can take on your body:

- **Mucolytic:** A mucolytic refers to a medicinal plant that helps break down and thin mucus to encourage its elimination. Mucolytic spices include horseradish, chili, and garlic. While mucus is protective, there can be a buildup of mucus, for example in the sinuses, which can become congested and cause pain.

- **Expectorant:** Expectorant spices are those that help the lungs, throat, and mouth expel mucus. They include chili and black pepper.
- **Antiviral:** Antiviral spices are those that help protect your body against viruses. Antiviral spices include licorice and ginger.
- **Demulcent:** Demulcent spices usually contain mucilages, which are soothing to the inner lining of your throat and esophagus. These types of spices can soothe mucous membranes and reduce inflammation. Spices that have these actions include licorice and cinnamon.
- **Antibacterial:** Some spices have antibacterial properties. Antibacterial spices can be useful for cuts and sore throats. Antibacterial spices include peppermint, thyme, garlic, horseradish, turmeric, and cinnamon.

Spices for the Immune System

As part of a healthy diet, spices can aid in keeping your immune system in tiptop shape, as they are both nutritious and can have therapeutic effects that can benefit your immune system. You already know that getting the right amount of vitamins and minerals is essential to good health, but keep in mind, you don't need to find these supplements in pills. Try your spice rack!

The Role of Spices in the Immune System

Spices have different actions and constituents that are applicable to the immune system. Spices have antimicrobial and antibacterial properties that are not merely for human benefit. The real reason some spices have these properties is due to each plant's biology, and these actions are actually mechanisms used to protect the plants. You can, however, take benefit of these properties to increase your health and support your immune system function.

Some spices can soothe the throat, some help break down mucus, and others can help reduce the severity of colds and flus. Spices can also help support the immune system through the foods they are cooked with, which will nourish you.

Supporting the Common Cold or Flu

Spices can be used acutely (and long term) to help ward off colds and flus and support your immune system. Spices with warming qualities are suitable to assist the body in the prevention and treatment of the common cold and influenza, especially in the cooler months. Warming spices also aid the removal of mucus, which is ideal for assisting the body in functioning well during cold and flu season. Warming spices include ginger, cardamom, and cinnamon.

Conditions That Spices Help Support

Spices may be used effectively to assist in supporting the body's immune system as well as with the following conditions:

- The common cold
- Influenza (the flu)
- Allergic rhinitis (hay fever)
- Sinusitis (inflammation in the sinuses)
- Upper respiratory tract infections (URTIs)
- Sore throat and coughing

Specific Spices for the Immune System

There are some spices that can directly help the immune system, for example medicinal spices that are antibacterial, antimicrobial, and antiviral. Others can add secondary benefits through certain properties that can soothe the throat and act more symptomatically.

Horseradish

Horseradish (*Armoracia rusticana*) is a root from the Brassicaceae (formerly Cruciferae) family. Horseradish is a great spice to help break down mucus in the sinuses. Horseradish has a pungent "spicy" taste.

Horseradish is a very hot spice and it can bring warmth to the extremities of the body. Horseradish can also be taken in supplement or tincture form, which can be prescribed by a qualified naturopath or herbalist, or can also just be eaten as part of the diet.

Thyme

Thyme (*Thymus vulgaris*) is such a common culinary garden plant, yet it is has many benefits, especially in the health of the immune system. Thyme contains the volatile oil thymol, which has been found in studies to be antibacterial. Traditionally thyme has been shown to have actions that are specific to the health of the throat and lungs, including being an expectorant, spasmolytic, antioxidant, and antimicrobial.

Onions

Onions (*Allium cepa*) have been used for thousands of years as a food and medicine. Onions are often used as a home remedy for colds and the flu, as a mucolytic plant. They also contain a prebiotic called fiber inulin, which is good for the immune system as it helps feed the good bacteria in your gut. There is an old remedy used for colds in which you place a cut-up onion in your bedroom overnight while you sleep or under the soles of your feet (and you wear socks over the top!). It is said to help reduce mucus and inflammation if you are suffering from a cold. Onions can of course be cooked in your meals to add flavor as well as their therapeutic properties. Some people experience abdominal discomfort eating onions due to the fermentable sugar they contain. If you experience this, you could substitute the green part of scallions instead.

Licorice

Licorice root (*Glycyrrhiza glabra*) is a plant commonly used in Western herbal medicine for treating hypothalamic-pituitary-adrenal (HPA) axis dysfunction or so-called "adrenal fatigue" and improving stress resilience. Licorice also has antiviral properties and is physically soothing to the mucous membranes. As it is antiviral it can be suitable for use during colds and flus. It is soothing to the throat because of its action as a demulcent and because of its constituents, the mucilaginous polysaccharides. In the 1800s, Mrs. Isabella Beeton mentioned in her book *Mrs. Beeton's Book of Household Management* a cold remedy recipe that included licorice root. The recipe was called "To Cure a Cold," and she said the remedy was to be taken "whenever the cough is troublesome." Little did Mrs. Beeton know just how effective and active licorice is for colds. Licorice has antiviral properties that are useful for colds and flus, as generally viruses contribute to these conditions, not only bacteria. Licorice can be made into a lovely tea, herbal cough drops, or into a syrup with honey to soothe your throat while you recover from a cold or from influenza. *Caution*: Licorice can increase blood pressure and has a cortisol sparing effect, so it is best to check with your healthcare provider to make sure this plant is suitable for you. Licorice should be used only short term and should be prescribed by a qualified herbalist.

Cinnamon Bark

"Cinnamon" can refer to a few varieties of the plant including true cinnamon (*Cinnamomum verum*) and Chinese cassia cinnamon (*Cinnamomum cassia*). Chinese cinnamon has a much stronger taste than true cinnamon, and generally Chinese cassia cinnamon is much cheaper in cost. True cinnamon is arguably the "healthier" version of cinnamon, as it does not contain the coumarins that Chinese cassia cinnamon does, which may be hepatotoxic (toxic to the liver) in large amounts. Cinnamon is astringent, mucilaginous, carminative, and an aromatic digestive that has a slightly sweet and bitter taste. You may notice if you eat cinnamon it can make your mouth feel a little dry; this is due to its astringent action and tannin content. Cinnamon is useful for colds and flus due to its antibacterial essential oils and its ability to form a mucilage, which is soothing to the mucosa. You can drink cinnamon in an infusion or decoction along with ginger and honey to taste.

 Alert

Never inhale cinnamon! Cinnamon is very toxic if you inhale it, so stick to using it in food and drink at recommended amounts.

Astragalus Root

Astragalus root (*Astragalus membranaceus*), also known as huang qi, is often used in food for its medicinal properties in traditional Chinese medicine, as well as in Western herbal medicine. Astragalus is a powerful immune booster and a tonic. It acts in the immune system by modulation of immune activity, and by its antioxidant function. You can find dried astragalus in Asian grocery stores and use it in your cooking, for example, in soups and stews. Astragalus can be cooked with other spices such as garlic, ginger, and onion as a synergistic immune-boosting combination. Astragalus should be avoided in the early stages of an infection and is better used preventatively.

Garlic

Garlic bulb (*Allium sativum*) is a well-known antimicrobial remedy and spice that has been used since ancient Egypt. According to the herbalist Maud Grieve, author of *A Modern Herbal*, garlic is diaphoretic, expectorant, diuretic, and a stimulant. Some cultures even avoid garlic due to its "stimulating" effect. Garlic has antioxidant and anti-inflammatory properties, too. These days, garlic isn't used to ward off beasts; it is, however, often used for infectious conditions, both topically and in food. It has been used in such conditions as ringworm and thrush due to its antimicrobial properties. Garlic can also help break down mucus due to its mucolytic action. It is also a great remedy for colds and the flu. This is because garlic contains allicin, which is the active, antimicrobial constituent. Garlic contains the constituent alliin, which after garlic is crushed or cut gets converted to allicin by the enzyme alliinase. Garlic needs to be exposed to air for about 10 minutes to release the allicin. Garlic can be taken in capsules (as prescribed by your qualified healthcare practitioner), eaten raw, used in salad dressings, and used in cooking.

Australian nutritionist Amanda Henham says that garlic "may be used as a 'tea' for acute infections with honey, lemon, ginger, cayenne pepper and apple cider vinegar. This is an excellent remedy for upper respiratory infections. Rich in manganese, vitamins B_1, B_6, and C, as well as selenium, copper, calcium, and phosphorus. Garlic is an excellent spice used in food as medicine for multiple conditions including the prevention of illness and disease. I use it daily in cooking to help keep the blood flowing and maintenance of the immune system. We experience far less frequent colds and flus than many families, even when serious and long-standing infections are prominent in the area." As with onion, garlic also contains oliogfructosaccharides, which may be problematic for some people.

 Fact

Did you know the reason you might get "garlic breath" is because some of garlic's constituents are excreted by the body via your lungs. You can help offset this aroma by eating a little bit of parsley or peppermint leaves, or by drinking peppermint tea.

Black Pepper

According to an article by researchers Murlidhar Meghwal and T.K. Goswami in 2012, black pepper (*Piper nigrum*), sometimes called the "king of spices," is an antioxidant, antipyretic (which means it helps reduce or prevent a fever), "anticancer," antiperiodic, antimicrobial, antibacterial, and an immune enhancer. It is thought to be an immune enhancer by "supporting the efficiency of white cells and assists the body to raise a powerful defense against invading microbes." It is also useful as an expectorant and mucolytic spice. Ground black pepper can be used on your daily meals. It can also be ground and mixed into honey as a remedy for coughs that present with a lot of mucus.

 Fact

Red "peppercorns" are not botanically related to *Piper nigrum*. What is sometimes included in pepper mixes along with black, white, and green peppercorns is in fact *Schinus terebinthifolius*.

Rose Petals and Rose Hips

According to a 2012 article by Hanan Youssef and Rasha Mousa in *Food and Public Health*, roses are antiviral and bactericidal. Rose hips and rose petals are a rich source of vitamin C, important for immune system health and well-being. Rose hip syrup is often used as a preventative treatment in winter months to ward off colds and flus. Rose petals are delicious additions to meals and can be consumed as a part of many dishes. You can try having a warm infusion of rose petals when you feel you are coming down with a cold or the flu.

Ginger

Ginger (*Zingiber officinale*) is an anti-inflammatory spice, suitable to the immune system. The rhizome or "root" is the part used therapeutically. According to research in the *Journal of Ethnopharmacology*, ginger may have antiviral properties. Ginger, in the form of tea, is also diaphoretic, meaning it can help raise your body temperature and keep you warm, as it increases sweating, which is ideal during times of low immunity, such as during a cold or flu. Ginger is best made into a warm infusion or decoction to enhance its warming and diaphoretic properties.

Chili

Chili (*Capsicum spp.*) is a spice that can help break down and thin excess mucus in the sinuses, and help the body get rid of it. The fruit and its encased seeds can both be used. Chili is diaphoretic as well. It is rich in vitamin C and very warming and stimulating. Chili is best used in very small amounts, due to its heating (and potentially burning) qualities. You can eat chili in soups and stews, casseroles, and broths, or a pinch can be added to tea.

Peppermint and Sage

Leaves from the peppermint plant (*Mentha piperita*) and common garden sage (*Salvia officinalis*) are antimicrobial and antibacterial. Both sage and peppermint can be used in mouthwashes, gargles, and to freshen breath. They can be used as herbal teas when you have a cold as well. Peppermint is diaphoretic, meaning it increases sweating and is naturally cooling, unlike the warming nature of other spices.

Myrrh

Myrrh (*Commiphora molmol*) can be a useful plant for the health of the mouth, as well as in the treatment of colds and flus. Myrrh is antiseptic, antimicrobial, antiparasitic, and anti-inflammatory. Traditionally it has been used to treat infections, respiratory conditions, respiratory catarrh, and for wounds, and also acts as an astringent, expectorant, and anticatarrhal. The *British*

Herbal Pharmacopoeia recommends myrrh for aphthous ulcers, pharyngitits, respiratory catarrh, and the common cold.

Fenugreek and Aniseed (Anise)

Aniseed (*Pimpinella anisum*) is an expectorant, which means it helps the body expel excess mucus out of the lungs. It is also an antispasmodic. Fenugreek (*Trigonella foenum-graecum*) is useful in the immune system as it is an expectorant, mucilaginous, and soothing to the mucous membranes, as a demulcent.

Olympic Gold Medalist, naturopath, and herbalist Lauren Burns says that "fenugreek (*Trigonella foenum-graecum*) or Kasuri Methi as it is often known, is an absolutely delightful herb. I frequently use both the dried seeds and leaves in my cooking. The leaves have a much more distinct and slightly bitter flavor, whereas the seeds offer a gentle aromatic warmth to the dish. I use the seeds in a base of most of my curries and dahl, making sure I heat them gently with other spices to remove bitterness. The leaves I tend to use more with a tomato base or curry containing root vegetables. I also use fenugreek when I am making idlis and fermenting the rice mixture. Add a pinch of fenugreek seeds to lentils as they are soaking. After this you blend the fermenting soaked rice and lentils until smooth. It then rests again before you make the lovely pillows of idli bread to mop up your curry of choice.

"Medicinally, fenugreek has been used traditionally as a galactagogue to assist milk production in breastfeeding mothers and to aid digestion. If you haven't cooked with fenugreek before I highly recommend trying it. The seeds in particular are a subtle yet fragrant aromatic."

Nigella Seed

The seed from the plant *Nigella sativa* is used in Ayurveda as a digestive, antiseptic, and as an overall tonic to aid healing. Nigella seed was even mentioned by Iranian philosopher Avicenna. Nigella has antibacterial, antifungal, antioxidant, and anti-inflammatory actions. *Nigella sativa* is thought to have properties that modulate the immune system, as well as those that help to reduce inflammation. According to an article in the *International Research Journal of Pharmacy* in 2011, Nigella seed contains thymoquinone, which is its main active constituent. Nigella's pharmacological properties may have some benefits as an analgesic, anti-inflammatory, antidiabetic, antimicrobial, and gastroprotective spice and herbal medicine.

CHAPTER 4

Spices for Inflammation

Inflammation is a protective biochemical process that happens when your immune system recognizes trauma or a foreign invader. While inflammation is usually a protective process, if it is chronic, it can become a problem because it can negatively affect the functioning of the body. If you find that you are struggling with inflammation in any part of your body, from your gut to your muscles or skin, you can lessen your body's inflammatory burden in many ways. Utilizing spices is one way you can help reduce inflammation, and you can do so just by including them in your daily diet.

What Is Inflammation?

Have you ever noticed when you have gotten a sore on your finger that it starts becoming red, sore, hot, and painful? These are some of the classic signs of inflammation. Inflammation is a part of the body's natural healing and protection system, the immune system. Inflammation is one of the body's first natural defense mechanisms. It is an important biochemical process as it aids in protecting the body from damage. Inflammation can happen as a consequence of infection, physical damage, deprivation of oxygen, poor nutrient supply, genetic or immune causes, as well as from chemicals and radiation.

The Problem with Inflammation

Inflammation is a necessary part of healing; however, an issue can arise when inflammation persists, when it becomes low grade, constant, and chronic. Chronic inflammation is inflammation that lasts longer than two weeks. This affects your body on a cellular, structural, and functional level. Inflammation affects the function of the organs or structure where the inflammation is present in the body. Inflammation can be found in a wide range of health conditions contributing to pain, edema, and joint stiffness. If you have inflamed tissues, you will generally know and you will feel it.

Causes of Inflammation

There is usually an underlying driver of inflammation. Your diet, your lifestyle, your stress levels, and the amount of exercise you get and the movements you make can potentially contribute to your body's inflammatory processes. Diet is particularly important, as many foods can have a pro-inflammatory effect on the body. Processed and refined foods that contain trans fatty acids and other fats and oils that have gone rancid may affect how your body handles and reduces inflammation. The good news is your diet can be modified to help your body produce more anti-inflammatory chemicals or mediators.

The Process of Inflammation

In order for inflammation to occur, first damage needs to happen in an area of the body; for example, a cut on your skin. After your body recognizes this damage, many immune cells are sent to ease the damage. With inflammation, you will first notice a vascular response, where you have an increased blood flow to the area of damage (which is why inflamed tissue is red) and swelling. Immune cells, called leukocytes, stick to blood vessel walls, while certain chemicals of inflammation, such as histamine, bradykinin, and prostaglandins, are released into the blood to the affected areas as a part of inflammation. Once inflammation occurs, its goal is to reduce damage and infection (if present), to control the process of inflammation, to help the adaptive immune system learn what is happening and help it become more efficient in the future, and to be clean and heal.

Certain plasma protein cell systems assist the process of inflammation. They are the complement, clotting, and the kinin systems. Inflammation is a very important healing process. When it goes awry, inflammation persists and is chronically present.

Inflammation and Health Issues

Inflammation is recognized in many disease processes and health conditions. These health conditions include obesity, type 2 diabetes, metabolic syndrome, heart disease, arthritic conditions, and mental health conditions. Talk to your doctor about what could be contributing to your inflammation. Here is a list of possible causes:

- Chronic stress
- Your diet
- Your environment
- Certain medications
- Toxic chemicals
- Low amounts of exercise and immobility

Obesity, Diabetes Mellitus (Type 2 Diabetes), and Heart Disease

According to Maria E. Ramos-Nino, in *International Scholarly Research Notices Oncology* in 2013, obesity is considered to be a condition of chronic inflammation caused by chemical reactions in the fat cells. Adipocytes (fat cells) have hormonal actions in the body. When the fat cells become enlarged, as in those who have become obese, they can encourage inflammation, due to an accumulation of macrophages (immune cells) and can upset insulin regulation.

Type 2 diabetes (diabetes mellitus) is a condition of insulin resistance in which the pancreas is unable to produce insulin from its beta cells. Inflammation can affect, or increase, the risk of diabetes through mechanisms including those that affect the adipose tissue cells. Researchers Eric Lontchi-Yimagou and Eugene Sobngwi believe that a certain kind of fat tissue, called white adipose tissue, is involved in these inflammatory processes. In this white adipose tissue, inflammatory cells are produced such as cytokines, and TNF-alpha, interleukin (IL) 1, IL-6, IL-10, and leptin.

Inflammation may be a driver in heart disease and atherosclerosis (the hardening of the arteries). Alex Dregan and Judith Charlton conclude in *Circulation* that the risk of cardiovascular diseases and type 2 diabetes is increased in those who have chronic conditions of inflammation.

⊖! Alert

Many skin conditions' pathophysiology involve inflammation. These skin conditions include eczema, dermatitis, and acne. Talk to your dermatologist about how to manage these conditions.

Metabolic Syndrome and Cancer

Metabolic syndrome is a collection of symptoms that includes abnormal levels of blood proteins, cholesterol, obesity, and high blood pressure that puts the body at a greater risk for cardiovascular disease and diabetes. Inflammation may be a driver in some types of obesity-associated cancers, according to researcher Maria E. Ramos-Nino. The National Cancer Institute (2015) states that inflammation is a risk factor for some types of cancers, including bowel cancer. They explain that "chronic inflammation may be caused by infections that don't go away, abnormal tissues, or conditions such as obesity. Over time, chronic inflammation can cause DNA damage and lead to cancer."

Mobility and Joint Health

The health of your joints can be affected when these joints and the muscles around them are inflamed. Pain is often a part of inflammation, which may make you less likely to exercise, which can make the issue worse. Common concerns that affect the joints include "-itis" conditions such as osteoarthritis, rheumatoid arthritis, ankylosing spondylitis, juvenile arthritis, bursitis, and gout, too. These conditions have a range of pathologies and causes. A diet of inflammatory foods may worsen these conditions and increase discomfort in the body.

Alert

Inflammation may affect certain gut conditions, sometimes by affecting the health of the gut's microbial population. Inflammation may be present in such conditions as inflammatory bowel disease (IBD), including Crohn's disease and ulcerative colitis.

Anti-Inflammatory Foods

Spices and quite a number of foods can have an impact on the inflammatory cascade in order to produce anti-inflammatory prostaglandins, which help reduce inflammation. You can manipulate your diet in a positive way by including many anti-inflammatory foods and spices. It can be as simple as including more fruits and vegetables and leaving out the most processed, refined, and sugary foods.

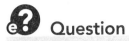 **Question**

How does inflammation affect your mental health?
Inflammation is thought to affect the disease processes of mental health conditions such as stress, depression, and anxiety. Stress can also produce inflammatory chemicals in the body. According to researchers George Slavich and Michael Irwin, a pathway in the brain may exist between stressors that occur in the social environment and inflammation. They also mention that there is a strong association in studies between stress and inflammation.

Anti-Inflammatory Diets

For a diet to be anti-inflammatory it may have:

- A good ratio of anti-inflammatory omega-3 fatty acids to omega-6 fatty acids. You generally want a higher proportion of omega-3 fats (found in fish and seafood, for example) to omega-6 fats (found in vegetable oils, such as corn oil).
- Anti-inflammatory foods such as a wide range of colorful fruits and vegetables, herbs, and spices.
- Limited processed and refined foods.

Lifestyle Factors to Help Reduce Inflammation

Sometimes looking at your lifestyle and addressing it can have a positive and holistic effect on reducing inflammation.

- **Rest and sleep:** Your body needs time to rest and repair, which is why getting enough sleep is so important to help reduce inflammation and keep your immune system healthy.
- **Exercise and movement:** When you exercise your body can break down inflammatory mediators and stress

chemicals. Movement is also important for your circulation to transfer blood, nutrients, and anti-inflammatory mediators around the body and to inflamed areas of the body.

- **Stress reduction:** Reducing stress is important for long-term management of inflammation, as well as the other benefits that go along with relaxation.

The good news is, reducing or modulating inflammation in the body is possible, and doing so may help with other ailments, including:

- Dysmenorrhea (period pain)
- Pain in the gastrointestinal tract (depending on the cause)
- Musculoskeletal disorders such as inflammatory conditions, e.g. osteoarthritis
- Stress
- Gastrointestinal conditions such as irritable bowel syndrome (IBS) and gastritis

Anti-Inflammatory Spices

Many spices have anti-inflammatory properties and constituents that help the body produce anti-inflammatory chemicals, called prostaglandins.

Turmeric

Turmeric (*Curcuma longa*) is the root that you know for its vibrant orange hue. Not only is turmeric delicious, but it can also help improve your health due to its highly anti-inflammatory properties. According to an article in the journal *Current Drug Targets* in 2011, turmeric, and its curcuminoids, have been found to reduce inflammation in gingivitis and to affect inflammation in conditions such as atherosclerosis, diabetes, and cancer, and conditions of the liver, gastrointestinal tract (especially intestinal and gastric conditions), the pancreas, respiratory system, neurons, and eyes. Turmeric may help reduce inflammation by inhibiting nuclear factor-kappaB, cyclooxygenase-2, and lipoxygenase, which normally promote inflammation.

Naturopath Helen Padarin asks, "What's not to love about turmeric? The golden spice, one of the most valuable medicinal spices in my mind, is so fantastic for liver function, anti-inflammatory activity and antioxidant activity that there is almost no health condition that does not benefit from consumption of turmeric."

Ginger

Ginger rhizome is traditionally used for its warming and anti-inflammatory properties. Ginger has been looked at in scientific studies to examine its potential to reduce inflammation. In cooking and tea mixes, ginger combines well with cinnamon, cloves, star anise, cardamom, and black pepper. It also is commonly cooked with garlic and onions. Ginger can be used as a food, as a spice, and as a tea.

Fresh Herbs

Many fresh herbs including rosemary, thyme, and oregano are thought to be anti-inflammatory due to their antioxidants and other phytochemicals and polyphenols. Fresh herbs can be included in your diet in many ways including as teas, and they can be added to salads, used to garnish meals, or even used as a base for a veggie-rich meal.

CHAPTER 5

Spices for Digestion

When you think of spices for health, you may think of how spices benefit your digestive system, and there is a good reason for this association. Spices can be added to your meals for not only their taste, but also their effect on your digestion, which can improve your overall health. Spices can aid your digestion by stimulating saliva and gastric acid production, soothing the stomach and gastrointestinal mucosa, and helping to relieve bloating, flatulence, and constipation. Spices are a key part of many cuisines, such as Indian, Thai, and Chinese, and their uses have both culinary and medicinal benefit. In fact, aniseed is often used as a digestive after meals in Indian restaurants.

The Importance of a Healthy Gut

You are more than just what you eat—you are what you absorb! What you know of as "the gut," the gastrointestinal tract is an amazing part of your digestive system. Your alimentary canal (the gut) spans from your mouth through to the end of your intestines, rectum, and ends with the anus. Only in recent years have researchers discovered how very important a healthy gut is to your overall health and well-being.

Issues in your gastrointestinal tract can affect digestive health through inadequate digestion and absorption, but it can affect the body as a whole as well. Gut dysfunction may affect the immune and nervous systems, the health of your skin, your mental focus and emotions, and contribute to food intolerances and inflammation. Your gut is interconnected with the rest of your body.

What Does the Gut Do?

A healthy digestive system does all the things you need it to do including, of course, digesting and absorbing your food, as well as playing a part in your immune system and your mental health. The following sections explain just how important your gut is to your overall health, and what it can do for the rest of your body.

In the Mouth

Your mouth is the first port of call for digestion. When you chew food in your mouth, you start to mechanically break it down with your teeth and also chemically with the enzyme salivary amylase, which helps break down carbohydrates and sugars. Your food next travels from your mouth to the stomach via esophageal muscular contractions, swallowing.

In the Stomach

Once your food has landed in your stomach, it is churned by the musculature of your stomach and is further broken down. Hydrochloric acid also assists digestion to chemically break down your food into smaller components.

The secretory cells in your stomach, the parietal and chief cells, produce substances such as mucus (which is protective to the stomach) and acid, hormones such as gastrin, enzymes, gastroferrin (needed for iron absorption), and intrinsic factor (needed for B_{12} absorption). Gastric acid has a protective function in your body, as it acts to break down your food. It also initiates the conversion of pepsinogen to pepsin, which is needed to break down proteins into smaller components, such as peptides. Gastric acid is also protective to your body through its ability to break down bacterial organisms and any incoming substances that land in your stomach. Your stomach also absorbs water, alcohol, copper, iodide, fluoride, and molybdenum. Some of these substances are important in the functioning and health of the body.

Accessory Digestive Organs

The accessory digestive organs support your body's main digestive organs by the products they produce.

- **The liver:** The liver produces bile, which is needed for emulsification of fats and lipids. The way fats and oils are emulsified by bile can be likened to how soap mixes with fats when washing dishes. Bile also helps digest dietary fats and lipids. The liver also helps transform your food into forms for storage later on, such as transforming glucose into glycogen (the storage form of glucose).
- **The gallbladder:** The gallbladder is your body's reservoir for bile. It is where bile lives until it needs to be released into the small intestine.
- **The pancreas:** The pancreas helps digest food by the enzymes it releases. Pancreatic enzymes include trypsin, pancreatic amylase, and lipase, needed for protein, carbohydrate, and fat absorption. The pancreas also produces insulin, which has a role in helping maintain blood sugar levels, and bicarbonate, which affects the pH of the body.

Small Intestine (SI): Duodenum, Jejunum, and Ileum

Next, your food, which is transformed into chyme, a mixture of partly digested food and stomach acid and other products, travels from your stomach and into your small intestine. The small intestine has three parts: the duodenum, the jejunum, and the ileum. The duodenum continues the physical breakdown of food. The small intestine also receives bile from the liver and pancreatic enzymes that continue digestion of proteins, carbohydrates, and fats. The small intestine also produces brush border enzymes, which also help break down the chyme into even smaller parts to be absorbed.

The duodenum, which is the first part of the small intestine, absorbs minerals such as calcium, phosphorus, magnesium, iron, copper, and selenium; the B vitamins thiamin (B_1), riboflavin (B_2), niacin (vitamin B_3); plus biotin, folate, and the fat-soluble vitamins A, D, E, and K. The jejunum, which is the second part of the small intestine, absorbs thiamin (B_1), riboflavin (B_2), niacin (B_3), pantothenate (B_5), biotin, folate, vitamin B_6, vitamin C, vitamins A, D, E, and K, as well as calcium, phosphorous, magnesium, iron, zinc, chromium, manganese, molybdenum, lipids, monosaccharides (simple sugars), amino acids, and small peptides (proteins). The last part of your small intestine, the ileum, absorbs vitamin C, folate, vitamin B_{12}, vitamin K, and magnesium along with bile salts and acids. Your small intestine, mostly the jejunum and ileum, is your body's nutritional absorption powerhouse.

The Large Intestine

Your large intestine is also a site of absorption, namely water, vitamin K, biotin, sodium, chloride, and potassium. Your large intestine also is very important as it produces short-chain fatty acids (SCFA). SCFAs are produced by your gut microbiota ("gut bugs") as a waste product from their digestion of fibrous foods. Diets that are high in fiber positively influence the microbiota's ability to produce more short-chain fatty acids. The main SCFAs produced by gut microbes include acetate, butyrate, and propionate. Most of the SCFAs are reabsorbed by the colon cells, while a small proportion of them are excreted with the feces. SCFAs may play a role in prevention in certain diseases such as metabolic syndrome, bowel disorders such as irritable bowel syndrome, and maybe even certain types of cancer. SCFAs are protective to your intestinal cells, are anti-inflammatory, and are an energy source for your colon cells.

The Immune System in Your Gut

Your gut is a protective barrier to the outside world and is a big part of your immune system. Your gut can actually be thought of as "outside" of your body, due to what it is exposed to.

For example, in the stomach, hydrochloric acid (stomach acid) acts as a chemical barrier and breaks down proteins and other substances such as bacteria. The inner lining in your intestine is a physical and chemical barrier. Your intestine is selectively permeable, which allows certain nutrients in and prevents invading microbes and large substances from entering. Your intestines contain specialized immune tissue, called the gut-associated lymphoid tissue (GALT). Examples of GALT include the tonsils and adenoids, Peyer's patches in the small intestine, the appendix, and lymphoid cells in your large intestine and rectum.

 Fact

Intestinal hyperpermeability: This occurs when the intestinal cells in your gut become "leaky," thus allowing certain things in that shouldn't normally be allowed to go through the gut lining. In intestinal hyperpermeability the intestinal cells can become inflamed and this can contribute to poor absorption, gastrointestinal symptoms, and systemic inflammation throughout the whole body.

Your Gut Is Home to Thousands of Microbial Allies

Bacteria are everywhere in and on your body, including on your skin and in the digestive tract. You actually have ten times more bacteria in and on your body than you have human cells! These microbes are not to be feared as they generally have a symbiotic and protective relationship with your body. Many even consider the gut microbiota, or microbiome, to be like an extra organ of the human body. The main bacteria that colonize your gut are Firmicutes, Bacteroidetes, Actinobacteria, Proteobacteria, Verrucomicrobia, Lentisphaerae, and Fusobacteria. Your gut can also be colonized with microbes other than bacteria, such as fungi.

You first receive the beginnings of your "gut microbiota" (that is, your gut microbes, collectively) when you are born, from the birth canal and also from breast milk and your environment. Most of your gut microbes are located in your large intestine. Certain bacteria play a protective role as a physical and chemical barrier in your intestines and as part of your immune system. Your microbiota also helps your immune system to learn and develop and act as a physical barrier to protect you from unwanted and unfriendly pathogens. They also produce antimicrobial factors and induce development of immunoglobulin A. Your gut microbes produce vitamin K and vitamin B_{12} and help regulate the motility of your gut. Your body helps provide food for your gut microbes through your dietary intake, mostly cellulose and other substances. The gut microbes also help transform many other dietary substances such as lignans and isoflavones into forms your body can use.

Alterations in microflora balance "good bugs" versus "bad bugs," also known as dysbiosis. Simon Carding and fellow authors report that dysbiosis of the gut has been linked with the pathogenesis of intestinal and extra-intestinal disorders. Extra-intestinal disorders are when other organs and systems of the body are secondarily affected by dysbiosis. Carding also explains that the conditions that are associated with dysbiosis (intestinal and extra-intestinal disorders) include inflammatory bowel disease (IBD), irritable bowel syndrome (IBS), celiac disease, metabolic conditions such as type 2 diabetes, allergy, autism, and other central nervous system disorders, along with asthma, cardiovascular disease, obesity, and colorectal cancer.

What can affect the health of your gut microbiome? Your levels of stress (mental, as well as physical), your diet (e.g., the amount of fiber you eat; if you consume antioxidant-rich or low-nutrient and refined foods), alcohol intake, antibiotic use, and cigarette smoke.

The Mind in Your Gut: "The Second Brain"

The gut has a strong connection to your brain, to your mental health, and to your emotions. The gut has even been referred to by Dr. Michael Gershon, a professor and researcher, as "the Second Brain." According to Gershon, the gut connects to your brain through the vagus nerve and your gut microbes. The vagus nerve, a cranial nerve that spans from your brain to your gut, functions independently from the rest of the body, so much so that if severed it still continues to function without the brain. The gut actually has its own nervous system as well, with the vagus nerve as a part of it; it is called the enteric nervous system (ENS).

 Fact

According to Kathryn McCance and Sue Huether (2010) your gastric secretions can be inhibited or increased by unpleasant odors and tastes, by pain, and also by emotions such as rage and fear.

Your gut microbes help the enteric nervous system to function and they influence neurotransmitter (brain chemical) production. The gut itself is thought to produce 80 percent of your body's own serotonin, the so-called "feel-good hormone." The combination of your gut microbes, your gut, the vagus nerve, and your brain has been termed the microbiota–gut–vagus–brain axis and simply the gut–brain axis. The gut–brain axis has been linked to skin conditions and mental health issues such as depression and anxiety.

Healthy Teeth and Gums

Good digestion really does start in the mouth, which requires healthy gums and teeth and good saliva production. Chewing and the release of saliva including the enzyme salivary amylase is important to effectively break down food. Certain spices may have a positive effect on the health of the gums and teeth.

Ginger

Ginger rhizome (*Zingiber officinale*) is a sialagogue, meaning it is an herb that can help stimulate saliva production. Ginger is also anti-inflammatory, antiviral, and antifungal and may be used as a mouthwash to help treat gingivitis.

Szechuan Pepper

Szechuan (or Sichuan) pepper berry, from the *Zanthoxylum* species, also stimulates saliva production. Adequate saliva production is required to digest your food and also for keeping your mouth, teeth, and gums healthy. When eaten, Szechuan pepper produces a tingling and numbing sensation in the mouth. This sensation is produced by a bioactive component called hydroxy-alpha-sanshool, an alkylamide. As a traditional spice, Szechuan pepper is thought to be a good remedy to help with toothache and facial pain that has originated from the trigeminal nerve, which is one of the twelve cranial nerves. Szechuan pepper is also delicious to cook with in many Chinese recipes.

Turmeric

Turmeric root (*Curcuma longa*) is commonly used in Ayurvedic medicine to keep the teeth and gums healthy. It is most likely able to do this due to its antibacterial and anti-inflammatory properties. The efficacy of turmeric, in the form of an oral gel, has been looked at in patients with severe gingivitis by H. Nilofer Farjana and S.C. Chandrasekaran. Ten subjects applied a turmeric gel to their mouths for twenty-one days. The researchers found a statistically significant result in this trial that showed the gel was effective in helping these patients to treat gingivitis due to a reduction of inflammation and bleeding. Toasted and ground turmeric preparations may also help reduce teeth pain and swelling in the mouth. It has also be used as a paste along with salt and mustard oil that is rubbed on the teeth and gums, and as a mouthwash for its bactericidal activity.

Peppermint and Chili

Peppermint (*Mentha piperita*) is an herb that contains menthol, a cooling and "fresh" smelling aromatic essential oil. Mint also contains antibacterial properties. Mint extracts are often used in toothpastes and preparations to cool and freshen the mouth. Menthol is thought to have this mouth-cooling effect through its ability to activate cold-sensitive somatosensory neurons.

Many varieties of chili (*Capsicum spp.*) may help stimulate saliva production as a sialagogue. Chili is also antimicrobial, antibacterial, and a strong circulatory stimulant. It is also rich in vitamin C and flavonoids.

Sage and Myrrh

Sage (*Salvia officinalis*) leaves can act naturally as an antibacterial herb and spice. Sage is often used in mouthwashes and to freshen the breath and can be included alongside mint as an herbal mouthwash.

The mystical myrrh (*Commiphora myrrha*) has antiseptic, antiparasitic, and anti-inflammatory actions. Some of the active constituents in myrrh include gums, resins, and volatile oils. Myrrh can be used as a mouthwash and can be used to treat and heal ulcers in the mouth.

Garlic and Clove

Garlic (*Allium sativum*) has been thought to be good for mouth ulcers. Garlic is another antimicrobial spice. Caution: garlic may cause burning in the mouth. Clove (*Syzygium aromaticum*), especially in the form of an essential oil, is a well-known home remedy for toothaches. A single clove may be chewed on to relieve toothache as well. The constituent eugenol is thought to be responsible for the pain-relieving action. Cloves also have antimicrobial properties, which could be indicated in certain oral conditions.

Improving Poor Digestion

Very often, people will continuously suffer with digestive problems, thinking that there is nothing they can do on their own to cure their ailments. While it is always helpful to receive a medical opinion and diagnosis for your digestive problems, you can also try using certain spices to ease your discomfort. Lucky for you, many spices are delicious, which makes improving your digestive system very easy.

Stimulating Digestion

Maud Grieve, author of *A Modern Herbal*, said of spices that "it has been well said, that the best quality of spices is to stimulate the appetite." Indeed, spices can improve one's appetite and digestion, thus improving health. You can help prepare your body for incoming food by eating or drinking certain spices that are bitter, sour, or have aromatic digestive properties, as they can stimulate your digestive functions. Spices may be suitable to stimulate appetite. The effect spices have on improving digestion is dependent on each spice's constituents, phytochemicals, and nutrients. Sometimes even just smelling certain spices may stimulate your saliva glands to produce saliva and stimulate your gastric acid secretions. Having a sense of hunger is a very important aspect of health, is a sign of vitality, and is one of the foundations of good health.

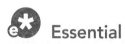 Essential

Dr. Ram Kishor Deshwal is an Ayurvedic doctor from Udaipur, Rajastan, India, who works to promote traditional Guni (the traditional healers) knowledge. According to Dr. Deshwal, spices that can help improve your digestion include long pepper (*Piper longum*), which is called *pippali* in Hindi; ginger (*Zingiber officinale*), called *saunth*; and asafetida, called *hing* (*Ferula asafoetida*), which is in the same family as allspice.

How Spices Help Stimulate Digestion

According to authors from the *Indian Journal of Medical Research*, Platel and Srinivasan (2004), spices have been hypothesized to aid digestion by stimulating the liver to secrete bile acids and by stimulating production of digestive enzymes, which are both important for healthy digestion. Spices can also be beneficial for digestive health by stimulating saliva release, increasing gastric acid secretions such as bile and hydrochloric acid, and increasing gastrointestinal absorption.

Warming Spices

Warming, aromatic spices are often used to increase digestive function. These spices include ginger, black pepper, cloves, cardamom, allspice, turmeric, cinnamon, and galangal.

Ginger

Ginger (*Zingiber officinale*) has a long history of being used as a digestion-enhancing herb and spice. It is a warming, aromatic digestive herb. Ginger has been used in many traditional medicine systems including in China, India, Iran, and Europe. Ginger is in the same family, Zingiberaceae, as turmeric and galangal. Ginger brings warmth to the body and the digestive tract, helping to increase blood supply to the digestive organs and the whole body, aiding in digestion, uptake, and assimilation of nutrients in the body.

Ajowan and Allspice

Ajowan is traditionally used to stimulate as well as soothe digestion. It is also used as a spice and flavoring in Indian curries. Ajowan has a flavor similar to that of thyme. Allspice is an aromatic spice that tastes similar to cloves. Allspice is a great herb to stimulate the digestive system, as a warming spice, as well as to calm and soothe the gut due to its carminative action.

Black Pepper

Black pepper has been traditionally used for expelling wind, reducing colic, increasing digestive function (especially when one has a cold constitution, meaning a tendency to feel cold), as well as heating the stomach. Pepper is naturally a "spicy" herb, which helps stimulate gastric acid and bring warmth to the body. Pepper may be used to aid in reducing constipation and diarrhea. Studies seem to suggest that black pepper may also be immunomodulatory, antioxidant, antiasthmatic, anticarcinogenic, anti-inflammatory, anti-ulcer, and have antiamoebic properties. Black pepper contains the alkaloid piperine. According to researcher Srinivasan (2007), piperine may exhibit effects that increase absorption in the digestive tract by stimulating pancreatic enzymes, affecting brush border enzymes, and reducing transit time in the gut. Piperine has also been examined by Meghwal and Goswami (2012) as a constituent that may protect against oxidative stress and damage, and it may also affect the bioavailability of certain drugs and plant constituents. Studies have shown that at various doses, pepper may have mild laxative effects, antisecretory and antidiarrheal activities, and may also have spasmodic and antispasmodic effects. Pepper is thought to help increase the absorption of other foods and spices, including turmeric. Maybe this ancient wisdom is why pepper is such a favorite on dinner tables.

Green Cardamom

In Indian Sanskrit texts *ela* means "cardamom." Green cardamom is often used as a spice in food and is an important part of the spice blend chai and as an ingredient in curries. Cardamom is a warming and slightly bitter spice. The herbalist David Hoffman describes cardamom as "carminative, sialagogue, orexigenic and aromatic." From these actions cardamom can be thought of as a spice that helps stimulate saliva production and increase appetite, and as an aromatic that can help reduce excess gas or flatulence in the gastrointestinal tract. Black cardamom is actually from a different plant than green cardamom; it comes from the plant *Amomum subulatum.*

Soothing the Gut

Spices can help soothe the gut in many ways. Spices can be used as infusions, which are essentially herbal teas, or decoctions, which are brews that require a longer simmer to soothe the gut. Spices can also be added to your meals, and as a bonus they help soothe your gastrointestinal mucosa and reduce bloating and flatulence after a heavy meal.

Common Symptoms and Conditions That Upset the Gut

Soothing the gut can refer to decreasing mucosal inflammation and discomfort along with reducing gastrointestinal symptoms such as cramps, abdominal pain, bloating, flatulence, hyperacidity, reflux, and diarrhea, and conditions such as irritable bowel syndrome.

Constipation is when your body has trouble releasing and excreting stools. Digestion is often sluggish as well. Certain spices can have a soothing effect on the gastrointestinal mucosa as well as helping to bind and move stools along the gastrointestinal tract. Spices that help bind stools are likely to do this because they can contain polysaccharides, which have a mucilaginous, slightly laxative effect. Mucilaginous herbs help decrease the time stools take to exit the gastrointestinal tract (i.e., bowel movements). They can do this by helping encourage peristalsis (bowel movements). They also contain fiber and mucilage content that helps to get things moving again and more regular.

Flatulence referrers to excess production of gas or wind in the stomach, intestine, and rectum and may also contribute to burping, bloating, and pain in the abdomen. Flatulence may be caused by food intolerances, low fiber intake as well as excess fiber intake, swallowing air, and poor digestion of foods and absorption issues.

For example, fermentable carbohydrates, known as FODMAPs, are known to cause flatulence in susceptible people. These foods include beans, onions, alcohol, dairy products, and starch-rich foods.

Bloating usually occurs due to food that has been poorly digested, microbial imbalances, from flatulence, "heavy" foods, refined foods, and food intolerances.

Spices to Soothe the Gut

Spices that help soothe the gut can be indicated in conditions such as constipation, flatulence, bloating, irritable bowel syndrome (IBS), gastric ulcers, and diarrhea. Some of the herbal/spice actions that help soothe the gut include antispasmodic, mucoprotective and anti-inflammatory, astringent, aromatic digestives, warming digestives, carminatives, mild laxative, stomachic, and spasmolytic. Specific spices that have gut-soothing actions include licorice, ginger, fennel, peppermint, fenugreek, cinnamon, dill, caraway, aniseed, coriander, cumin, and asafetida.

Ginger

Ginger has traditionally been used in gastrointestinal complaints due to its actions as an aromatic, warming digestive and antispasmodic herb and spice. Ginger has been found to be able to stimulate gastric emptying and contractions in the stomach in those who have functional dyspepsia. Ginger is also suitable for flatulence and may help in preventing constipation. Ginger may possibly act as an agent against *H. pylori*, a type of bacteria.

Ginger contains many constituents including volatile oils (that consist of monoterpenes and sesquiterpenes). The pungent taste of fresh gingerroot is due to its gingerol content. Dried ginger contains more shogaol, as the drying action causes the gingerol to convert into shogaol. Gingergol has a more pungent taste while shogaol has a spicier flavor, which is why dried and fresh ginger taste different and can be used differently.

Licorice

The root of licorice, *Glycyrrhiza glabra*, is another mucilaginous herb that can be used to improve the health of the gut. Licorice can be used in conditions of hyperacidity or gastrointestinal ulcers, due to the root's mucilaginous properties. The mucilage helps with these conditions as it soothes the gastrointestinal lining and reduces inflammation. Licorice is a spice that is protective to the mucosal linings.

Helicobacter pylori (*H. pylori*), a pathogenic bacterium, is often the cause of gastrointestinal ulcers, due to its ability to burrow into the gastrointestinal lining of the stomach. In a double-blind, placebo-controlled study by Sreenivasulu Puram, Hyung Chae Suh, and co-authors in 2013, the researchers looked at the effects of the deglycyrrhizinated form of licorice root extract on *H. pylori* infection. The deglycyrrhizinated licorice root is an extract that has had the glycyrrhizin portion removed. This constituent is known to increase blood pressure, which is why it is removed. Herbalists may use a deglycyrrhizinated form of licorice (DGL) in certain gastrointestinal conditions. In this study, there was a placebo and a treatment group, and all subjects tested positive for *H. pylori*. For sixty days, the treatment group were given 150 mg of the standardized deglycyrrhizinated *Glycyrrhiza glabra* extract. After sixty days, there was a statistical difference between the treatment group and the placebo group, with the treatment group showing a reduction in *H. pylori*. Apart from licorice's therapeutic uses, it can be added to food, drinks, and confections as a flavoring agent, though it should be cautioned in those with high blood pressure, so always discuss with your doctor if you plan to take any form of licorice root, be it in food or as a supplement.

Fenugreek

Not only is fenugreek seed a very flavorful spice, but it also may help your body reduce constipation. One of the constituents of fenugreek includes mucilage. Mucilage is a "slimy," gel-like substance that forms when it comes in contact with water. This is much like what forms from linseeds when they are soaked in water. This mucilage helps soothe the gastrointestinal tract and its mucous membranes. Mucilaginous plants also help soothe the stomach by protecting the stomach lining. This mucilage can also help reduce constipation as it helps bulk the stools. It is important to drink more water when using mucilaginous herbs or spices. In traditional herbal medicine fenugreek is also used as a galactagogue, a substance that helps encourage breast milk production in nursing mothers.

Cinnamon and Fennel

Cinnamon is an aromatic and warming digestive herb. It is a slightly bitter herb that is also mucilaginous and astringent. Astringent herbs and spices may be useful as an adjunct treatment in diarrhea.

Fennel (*Foeniculum vulgare*) is often mentioned as a spice and herb to help reduce flatulence because of its antispasmodic and carminative actions. Many parts of fennel can be used to aid in reducing flatulence. The seeds can be crushed and used in cooking. They can also be added to hot water for a refreshing, flatulence-busting tea. The bulb, stems, and leaves can also be cooked or they can be eaten raw, for example in salads. Fennel has an anise-like taste, which some may find quite pleasant and easy to cook with and consume.

Aniseed and Caraway

Aniseed, also known as anise, is an aromatic spice that helps reduce spasms in the gastrointestinal tract. It is also carminative and thought to be antiparasitic. Anise can be chewed at the end of a meal as a carminative spice to soothe the gut.

Caraway seed (*Carum carvi*) is also carminative, aromatic, and astringent, so it could potentially be used to reduce diarrhea.

Peppermint

Peppermint (*Mentha piperita*) is cooling and refreshing. The mint leaves are carminative, an action that helps soothe the digestive system.

Peppermint also possesses antiemetic (nausea-reducing), antiseptic, antispasmodic, and antimicrobial actions. It may help reduce abdominal pain as an analgesic and can be helpful for indigestion. Mint is a great herb that is often used in the symptomatic treatment of irritable bowel syndrome (IBS). IBS is a condition in which the microbiota can be altered from dysbiosis, or small intestinal bacterial overgrowth (SIBO). In an in vitro study by Thompson and Meah in 2013, essential oils of mint were looked at against *Escherichia coli*. The authors of the study found that peppermint essential oils, along with coriander seed oils, were quite potent and exhibited antibacterial activity. Peppermint oil is often found as enteric-coated forms and dosage is best advised by your healthcare practitioner. After-dinner mints are often served at the end of a meal to help soothe digestive function and reduce indigestion. Peppermint should be avoided by those with gastroesophageal reflux disease or heartburn issues, as it can relax the lower esophageal sphincter, which allows gastric acid up the esophagus.

Dill and Galangal

Dill seed (*Anethum graveolens*) is a spice and herb that has antispasmodic, carminative, and stomachic actions. The German Commission E recommends dill for dyspepsia.

Galangal (*Alpinia galanga*) is a carminative rhizome, which helps reduce flatulence.

Coriander

Coriander seed (*Coriandrum sativum*) can be used as a spice to help reduce excess gas in the gastrointestinal tract and to help lessen muscular contractions and spasms in the gut as well.

Coriander is antispamodic and antimicrobial. Coriander leaves, stems, and roots are often used in cooking and in salads to add a fresh hit of flavor. Coriander has been trialed along with lemon balm and peppermint to see whether they have antimicrobial actions in IBS. Coriander showed strong antimicrobial actions along with the peppermint. Coriander leaves, stems, and roots are also thought to have a detoxifying effect in the body.

Garlic and Star Anise

Herbalist Nicholas Culpeper believed that garlic, *Allium sativum*, "expels wind." Star anise is often used as an ingredient in Chinese cooking and in stocks. Star anise has carminative, stimulant, and diuretic actions. According to herbalist Matthew Wood, "the oil or a decoction or tincture is used as a sweet, warm, pungent, carminative, antispasmodic . . . ." These actions are particularly indicated for soothing and calming the gastrointestinal system.

Cumin

Traditional medicine systems of Iran, Tunisia, and India all use cumin (*Cuminum cyminum*), and it is thought to have antidiarrheal effects. Cumin's affect on rats has been studied by Himanshu Bhusan Sahoo and Saroj Kumar Sahoo et al. (2014) to determine whether an extract of this spice is useful in diarrhea. The result of the study showed that the aqueous solution of cumin has a significant effect on the frequency of diarrhea, reducing it along with defecation time, and slowing down the secretion of intestinal fluid and propulsion.

Asafetida

Asafetida is an oleo gum resin that is useful in the gastrointestinal tract, as it is an antispasmodic spice and a digestive aid. It has been used to help with "hysteria," nervous conditions, bronchitis, asthma, and whooping cough, and as an expectorant, stimulant, emmenagogue, vermifuge, and as a sedative. Asafetida oleo gum resin may be used as a substitute for garlic or onion in recipes, as it is FODMAP-free. According to Poonam Mahendra and Shradha Bisht (2012), asafetida may be a good remedy for gastrointestinal conditions such as flatulence, distention of the stomach, and gastric ulcers, and has been shown to increase pancreatic lipase, amylase, and chymotrypsin, in a rat study. Asafetida is also used in Krishna cooking, as devotees of this religion do not consume onions and garlic.

Keeping Your Liver Healthy

Your liver does so much for your body and can be a much underappreciated and neglected organ. Having a healthy liver is important for whole-body health as the liver performs hundreds of functions to keep your body healthy every single day.

What Does Your Liver Do?

Your liver performs a number of metabolic and biochemical actions. These actions include (and are not limited to) the following:

- The liver produces bile. Bile is one way your body excretes metabolic wastes. Bile helps emulsify and digest fatty acids and it also helps lubricate your bowels, which is important for keeping your bowel movements regular and to reduce constipation.
- The liver detoxifies chemicals and drugs, such as ammonia and alcohol, and other substances.
- The liver transforms pharmaceutical drugs into forms your body can use properly.
- The liver transforms food (such as proteins, fats, and carbohydrates) into usable forms for your body to use as energy.

- The liver breaks down the storage form of glucose so your body can use it, and it helps regulate glucose.
- The liver stores vitamins (such as vitamins D, K, and A, and B_{12}) and minerals (such as iron).
- The liver can produce nutrients for itself as well as for the whole body.
- The liver produces cholesterol needed for hormone production.
- The liver is a storage site for blood.
- The liver breaks down hormones and helps excrete them.

How the Liver Detoxifies

"Liver detoxification" is such a buzzword. Although liver detoxification seems to be used in many fad diets, there is a lot of merit to improving your liver function and its detoxification processes. You can definitely benefit from having a healthier liver. Naturopaths and integrative practitioners may associate poor liver detoxification with a number of conditions including menstrual and hormonal complaints, chemical sensitivities, skin conditions, headaches, pain, gastrointestinal conditions, and conditions of the immune system. The liver has a number of detoxification pathways. There are two main phases of liver detoxification, phase 1 and phase 2. Certain foods, herbs and spices, and substances can activate or inhibit certain phases of liver detoxification as well.

Phase 1 Liver Detoxification: Modification and Biotransformation

The first phase of liver detoxification involves modification and biotransformation of substances by the cytochrome P450 enzymes.

The cytochrome P450 are important for the detoxification of drugs, xenobiotics, and xenoestrogens, which are environmental estrogens. Phase 1 also metabolizes steroid hormones. Phase 1 actually makes the substances slightly more toxic, until they are conjugated in phase 2. This phase breaks down substances to turn them from fat-soluble into water-soluble and then they are sent off to phase 2 for conjugation. Phase 1 involves the biotransformation of substances by three processes: oxidation, reduction, and hydrolysis.

Phase 1 can be activated by cigarette smoke, green tea, and alcohol. Phase 1 can be inhibited by carrageen, certain drugs, and grapefruit juice (this is why it is generally recommended to be avoided with certain pharmaceutical drugs). Furthermore, Romilly E. Hodges and Deanna M. Minich describe herbs, spices, and other foods that induce and inhibit phases 1 and 2. Phase 1 includes rosemary, garlic, green tea, and cumin. DeAnn Liska (1998) explains nutrients required for phase 1 and 2 detoxification include riboflavin (vitamin B_2), niacin (vitamin B_3), pyridoxine (vitamin B_6), folic acid, vitamin B_{12}, glutathione, branched-chain amino acids, flavonoids, and phospholipids.

Phase 2 Liver Detoxification: Conjugation

Conjugation in phase 2 of liver detoxification involves a number of enzymatic processes. Conjugation is basically when certain molecules in your body are attached to a link on a drug or other substance. Conjugation processes include glucuronidation, acetylation, sulfation, glutathione conjugation, and amino acid conjugation.

Dietary factors can affect these phases. Phase 2 can be activated by cruciferous vegetables, certain herbs, spices, and nutrients. Phase 2 can be inhibited by nutritional deficiencies, poor diet, and certain medications.

Specific nutrients are important for phase 2 liver detoxification. These include specific amino acids (such as glycine and taurine) found in protein-rich foods, and also B vitamins, vitamin A, vitamin C, magnesium, zinc, selenium, and chromium.

Amino acids and glutathione are used in phase 2 conjugation reactions, as Dr. Mark Percival reveals (1997). Spices and vegetables such as onions, garlic, and vegetables such as cruciferous vegetables (broccoli and cabbage), help to support liver detoxification as well.

In a nutshell, your liver aims to break down substances into fat-soluble substances to be excreted into your bowels and water-soluble ones to be excreted by your kidneys. Your kidneys and bowels need to be working well to help your body get rid of these wastes.

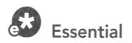 **Essential**

After your liver detoxifies and metabolizes certain substances, they need to be removed from the body. The wastes are usually sent to be excreted in the bile or are released by the kidneys as a part of urine. This process is known as excretion.

What Can Make Your Liver Unhealthy?

There are a variety of substances that can compromise the health of your liver. The following list details only a few:

- **Excess alcohol:** Alcohol can contribute to nutritional deficiencies as well as affect the health of the liver cells, the hepatocytes. Alcohol also affects the liver's own ability to detoxify from alcohol consumption.
- **Excess carbohydrates and a high-caloric/sugar diet:** Non-alcoholic fatty liver disease (NAFLD) is a form of liver disease that is thought to be worsened by a hypercaloric diet that is rich in trans and saturated fatty acids, cholesterol, and fructose-sweetened beverages, according to researchers Fan and Cao (2013), in the *Journal of Gastroenterology and Hepatology*.
- **Fatty liver disease:** Fatty liver disease can be nonalcohol induced and alcohol induced.

- **Certain medications:** Some medications can contribute to drug-induced liver damage such as acetaminophen, amoxicillin/clavulanate, isoniazid, and nonsteroidal antiinflammatory drugs (NSAIDs). Herbal and nutritional supplements, if not monitored correctly and if they are of poor quality, may also negatively affect the health of the liver. It is best to check with your doctor before taking any new medication and to read all labels on any medication you buy over the counter.
- **Poor diet:** A diet low in nutritious foods and high in processed and refined foods can cause damage to your liver as you may not be receiving enough nutrients and protective phytochemicals to help protect your liver and keep it functioning well.
- **Genetic differences:** For some people with genetic mutations, liver function and metabolic processes may be altered.

Dietary Approaches to Keep Your Liver Healthy

The following is a list of foods that can help keep your liver healthy. Try to incorporate these foods into your daily diet for best results:

- Bitter foods such as dandelion root and bitter green vegetables. Bitter foods are traditionally used to increase digestive function and are thought to help to stimulate bile production and release from the liver.
- Protein-rich foods from animal proteins such as chicken, eggs, beef, or protein-rich sources from plants such as legumes, beans, nuts, and seeds. Certain amino acids are important for liver detoxification and repair.
- As a food and an herbal extract, globe artichoke is traditionally used to improve liver detoxification.
- Sulfur-rich foods such as garlic and onions.

Spices (and Herbs) for a Healthy Liver

You can encourage your liver to gently continue its detoxification duties by including certain foods, spices, and herbs in your diet. Herbs and spices can have a protective influence on the liver and improve its detoxification efficiency. Some spices may activate different phases of liver detoxification including caraway, ginger, garlic, turmeric, rosemary, sage, and dill. Your liver is also important for your body to transform spice constituents into forms that your body can use.

Garlic and Turmeric

Garlic (*Allium sativum*) contains sulfur compounds. Sulfur is used to stimulate the various pathways in the liver, including phase 2 liver detoxification and pathways that affect carcinogens.

Turmeric (*Curcuma longa*) is thought to be protective to the liver as a hepatoprotective spice and an antioxidant-rich rhizome. Turmeric is also thought to be a spice that affects liver detoxification. Turmeric is protective to the liver and it is a phase 2 detoxifier.

Rosemary

Rosemary (*Rosmarinus officinalis*) is a well-loved herb in roasts, soups, and stews. While rosemary is more of an herb than a spice, it is worth including in this section. The part we use is the rosemary leaves, which are aromatic and originate from the *Rosmarinus officinalis* plant. Rosemary is a plant that protects the liver, termed hepatoprotective in herbal medicine. Its hepatoprotective actions may be due to its essential oil content. According to Aleksandar Rašković and Isidora Milanović (2014), rosemary's essential oils contain the main constituents cineole, camphor, and alpha-pinene. Rosemary also contains carnosol, carnosic acid, ursolic acid, diterpenes, rosmarinic acid, and caffeic acid, some of which are thought to contribute to rosemary's antioxidant properties. Rosemary is thought to work on activating phase 2 liver detoxification.

Green Tea

Although not typically thought of as a spice, green tea deserves an honorable mention. Many parts of the *Camellia sinensis* plant are used and processed in different ways to produce black tea, green tea, and white tea. Green tea can be processed in a variety of ways to create many types of green tea. Green tea contains catechins, which are antioxidants, such as epigallocatechin-3-gallate. These catechins may have a positive effect on liver detoxification.

Simple Nutritional and Exercise Tips for a Healthy Gut

There are some things that you can generally do to improve your digestive function. You can improve the quality of your diet, make sure you are well hydrated, and look after your emotional health. You can also improve your digestion by:

- **Addressing any nutritional deficiencies.** You need certain nutrients for a healthy digestive system. These nutrients include iron and zinc, which are needed to produce hydrochloric acid. Protein-rich foods are also important for healthy digestive function as they are needed in liver detoxification processes and for forming new cells in the gastrointestinal lining.
- **Addressing any food intolerances or allergies.** For example, those with celiac disease need to avoid gluten-containing foods and grains, as do those with non-celiac gluten sensitivity. Avoiding foods that are you are sensitive to is important if they continue to cause you issues, but this can be properly assessed with your qualified healthcare practitioner.
- **Drinking enough water.** Water helps soften your stools and helps makes them easier to pass. With regular, easier

to pass bowel movements, you will have a better functioning gastrointestinal tract.

- **Eating fibrous foods.** You need to eat enough fibrous food and have a balance of the right types of fiber: soluble and insoluble fibers. Soluble fiber comes from such foods as lentils and beans, psyllium husks, oats, nuts and seeds, and fruits such as apples, oranges, and pears. Insoluble fiber comes from vegetables and grain products. Fiber acts as an intestinal broom by sloughing off dead cells in the gastrointestinal tract and by taking excess hormones with it (in bile) on the way out. Fiber also helps keep your bowel movements regular and can reduce constipation.
- **Eating prebiotic and probiotic foods.** You can help encourage healthy microbial populations in your gastrointestinal tract by eating prebiotic and probiotic foods, which help feed your gut bugs. Prebiotic foods are those that help feed and nourish the gastrointestinal microbiota. Garlic and onion are prebiotics, as well as legumes, beans, and certain kinds of starches. Probiotic foods include sauerkraut, kimchi, and yogurt.
- **Eating protein-rich foods.** Protein-rich foods are important for healing, building, and repair in the gastrointestinal tract, as they are important building blocks in the body. Amino acids, the smaller components of proteins, such as glutamine also play a role in strengthening the gut wall.
- **Exercising.** You need to get enough daily movement and exercise to keep your bowels moving. Physical exercise helps to tone the bowel and keep it functioning well.
- **Reducing stress.** Managing and reducing stress is important for long-term gut health management. Stress can affect the health of your microbiota as well. You may have noticed feeling butterflies in your stomach or felt anxious and noticed symptoms in your gut; this feeling is due to your enteric nervous system (ENS) at play. Your

ENS and your emotions can affect the motility and activities of your gastrointestinal tract. Improving your stress tolerance may have a positive impact on gastrointestinal symptoms and mental health.

- **Avoiding antibiotics, except when absolutely necessary.** Antibiotics are an important, lifesaving medicine class; however, they can have a negative effect on the microbiome by destroying microbes, not only the bad microbes but the good ones as well, and this is why antibiotics are needed only in certain cases. Avoid taking antibiotics when you have a cold, since colds are caused by viruses, not bacteria (which antibiotics target). It is important to finish the course of antibiotics when you are on them and to follow your doctor's instructions. If you are taking antibiotics, you may benefit from consuming prebiotic foods and taking a probiotic supplement. Note: it is important to take the probiotic supplements at least two hours away from antibiotics.

Caution for Spices in the Gastrointestinal System

Some spices are contraindicated in certain gastrointestinal conditions and certain health conditions. These contraindications and cautions include:

- Those who are intolerant to FODMAPs. FODMAPs stands for fermentable, oligosaccharides, disaccharides, monosaccharides, and polyols. For some people these are hard to absorb. Those who are intolerant to FODMAPs may notice bloating and flatulence if they consume these foods. Instead of onion or garlic you can try asafetida in your cooking, which is free of FODMAPs.

- Some spices may increase symptoms of heartburn in those who suffer from it.
- Spices may be contraindicated in those with peptic ulcers.
- Spices may be cautioned in those with very sensitive digestions.
- Keeping it simple with spices and not including too many spices or too much can also be better for certain people if they have sensitive digestive function.
- Having too much spice, especially chili, may cause unpleasant gastrointestinal effects such as nausea and diarrhea.

CHAPTER 6

Spices for Brain Health, Better Cognition, and Happiness

Some of the most common mental health issues include stress, depression, and anxiety. There is much one can do to manage and lessen the impact of these conditions from a nutritional perspective. Maintaining brain health requires a holistic approach. Holistic health is looking at a variety of ways to improve and maintain one's health and the whole body. This can be done by looking after your diet, improving your self-care, resting, finding and maintaining nurturing relationships, and exercising.

Brain Health, Better Cognition, and Happiness

Mental health issues are something we are faced with often these days. Your brain and mental health are interlinked in your human physiology. Brain health is essential for your well-being due to its function as the controller of your body. Your brain is responsible for the generation of thoughts, your memories and retention of information, your moods and emotions, and your cognition.

Good Mental Health

Mental health is more than just how you think. Good mental health is about attending to your health and being proactive, rather than neglecting your health. Your mental health and state of well-being is very individual. Mental health conditions can be multifaceted and complex. They can involve complex pathophysiologies, and in the case of mental health issues, complex pathologies.

What Can Affect Brain and Mental Health?

There are many factors involved in mental health issues and brain pathologies, and the issues can be more than just what is happening in your brain. Issues can stem from elsewhere in the body.

The factors include:

- Inflammation in the body, especially the brain
- Any illnesses that affects the brain
- Your levels of stress
- Past experiences of emotional trauma
- A diet that contains low-nutrient foods
- Low amounts of movement and exercise
- The amount of water you drink
- Alcohol abuse
- Drug use, including illicit drugs
- The health of your gut, its digestive capacity, and your gut microbiota
- Your neurotransmitter production
- How well you sleep and whether you get enough sleep
- Physical damage to your brain
- Conditions of cognitive decline
- Your genetic expression
- Other physiological conditions

As you can see, there are many factors that can affect the brain and mental health, so sometimes mental issues and addressing them aren't so simple.

How Stress Affects Your Brain Health

There is a pandemic of stress in the modern world. You know what stress feels like for you. It can be purely a feeling in your mind, or you may experience it as an uncomfortable or uneasy feeling in your gut. It may feel like tight, tense shoulders and muscles, or you might even notice that you are stressed and a racing mind affects how you sleep at night. You may also feel that you are quite prone to stress and that you are a very stressed person. Stress is all very individual and you may find that addressing stress is quite difficult at first; however, there are many ways to address stress and make it less of a burden on your life.

Eustress versus Distress

Some amount of stress is necessary in your day-to-day life. It is important to your health and helps you get things done. This kind of stress is called eustress. Distress is the more negative form of stress, which is prolonged.

General Adaptation Syndrome (GAS)

The theory of GAS was originally put forward by Dr. Hans Selye. These stages are used to gauge and categorize stress. Kathryn McCance and Sue Huether (2010) describe the three main stages of stress, called general adaptation syndrome. In this three-step process, there is an **alarm stage** (where the central nervous system is stimulated and your body's defenses are mobilized), a stage of **resistance** (or **adaptation**) (where the mobilization activates fight-or-flight mode), and then there is the stage of **exhaustion** (where ongoing stress breaks down the compensatory mechanisms and balance of the body).

The Biological Process of Stress

Any way you experience stress, whether it is physical, emotional, or psychological, produces the same stress hormones in your body. Stress, as a biological process, starts when your brain is stimulated by a stressor, that is, anything that causes stress. This stressor then stimulates hormones in your brain such as corticotropin-releasing hormone (CRH), which go on to stimulate other hormones and produce other effects. Your limbic (emotional) system is stimulated by stress and releases the fight-or-flight stress hormone and neurotransmitter, norepinephrine, which gives your body the typical feelings of stress such as increased blood pressure, an increase of blood flow to muscles, pupil dilation, sweating, and makes you more adept at handling stress at the present moment. CRH stimulates antidiuretic hormone (ADH), which prevents you from urinating temporarily (important if you need to run away). Oxytocin, prolactin, endorphins, growth hormone, and adrenocorticotropic hormone (ACTH) are also stimulated and released. Dr. Sara Gottfried says that the "adrenal glands sit like hats on [y]our kidneys."

A specific part of the adrenal glands, called the adrenal medulla, releases hormones, called catecholamines. These hormones are called epinephrine and norepinephrine. Epinephrine affects cardiac function by increasing the heart's contractions, it increases the heart rate and blood pressure, and it dilates the blood vessels, causing greater blood flow to your muscles. It also increases your blood sugar levels.

Cortisol is released by the adrenal cortex, the other part of your adrenal glands, during stress. Cortisol stimulates the production of energy and helps with how protein is synthesized in the liver, which is important as stress breaks down protein in other areas of the body. Cortisol also stimulates the production of fats, which in the long term may contribute to obesity. You can imagine as cavemen and women we would need these adrenal hormones to help us run from predatory beasts. These days you might not deal so much with physical beasts as you may with the more psychological "beasts" that come up in everyday life and its ongoing associated stressors.

The Impact of Stress

Unfortunately with chronic stress there are repercussions and far-reaching systemic effects. Sayings such as "pulling your hair out with stress" often does ring true in a chronically stressed person. Stress can affect how well your body uses nutrients, and it uses up reserves of antioxidants, impacting the health of your body overall. It is a drain on your mind and on your body. Stress has the potential to affect your immune system, your hormonal system, your emotions, your cardiovascular health, your muscular health and tone, and the health of your gastrointestinal tract.

Self-Care Routines

Finding ways to deal with and reduce stress is important to your well-being. Thankfully nutritional medicine, herbal medicine, massage, and other physical therapies, as well as other holistic modalities such as counseling, offer many solutions to help you reduce stress and improve your stress tolerance. These modalities and therapies may also help you change how you react to stress, how you tolerate stress, and help you relax your mind.

What Is Self-Care?

Self-care is the act of looking after yourself emotionally, mentally, and physically. Self-care should be a priority in your life to have a healthier, happier body and mind. When you actively aim to reduce a negative stress response, it can help calm your mind and your nervous system.

Here are some suggestions for more self-care:

- Make a little time, every day, to relax—whether it is fifteen minutes, a day, or longer. Relaxing can be as simple as taking a few moments to take some long, deep breaths.
- Spend less time on social media, and more time interacting with people face to face. These days people often seem more "connected" with their computers than they are with actual people.
- Try writing. Write down your thoughts. Often it can be easier to process your thoughts when you have written them down.
- Watch your self-talk. What you think and say to yourself matters. This is because your thoughts form the basis of how you feel about yourself and the development of your own self-image.
- Set an exercise schedule. Regular exercise increases endorphins and muscular tone not only in your musculature but in your digestive tract as well, which helps you feel happier. Exercise also helps break down stress and inflammatory mediators.
- Deep abdominal (or yogic) breathing can be very beneficial to help quiet the mind and make you feel much more relaxed. This will also help improve your oxygen intake.
- Getting enough sleep is important for stress management. If you don't have enough sleep, your body cannot rest fully and this will affect your ability to handle stress properly.

Resilience, Better Moods, and Less Stress

How you act in life, how you think, and how resilient you are can affect your stress levels and your moods. Happiness and living a happier life is very individual. Happiness can be obtaining a good balance between life, work, family, and relationships. It can be about engaging in life and in the world and being proactive in fulfilling your goals and wants in life. Being positive, engaging in the world, and taking time to relax and enjoy life are all good approaches to living a happier, healthier life.

Foods for Brain Health and Happier Moods

There are simple ways you can modify your diet to make it more energy and mood sustaining, which may also help with managing your stress levels.

You need a balanced diet for optimal neurotransmitter production and stable blood sugar levels. Your blood sugar levels can have an influence on your moods and emotions.

FOODS THAT WON'T ENCOURAGE HEALTHIER MOODS

- Foods high in sugar: These will sap your energy and can affect your moods negatively.
- Processed and refined foods: These foods are low in the nutrients your body needs to produce and sustain energy and for healthy moods.
- Low-protein foods: Eating a diet that is rich in carbohydrate-rich foods may mean you are not eating enough protein. Protein-rich foods may help support healthier moods as they can help you to feel full and nourished.

Foods to Stock Up On
The following is a list of specific types of foods that will help promote brain health:

Protein-rich foods: Protein is needed for neurotransmitter (brain chemical) production. Amino acids are the building blocks for proteins. Certain amino acids are important for the production of these neurotransmitters, including glycine, glutamate, and proline. Protein comes from many foods, but is much more bioavailable in animal proteins such as meat, eggs, chicken, dairy, and seafood. Sources that have less protein bioavailability include soy products, legumes, nuts, and seeds. Protein also helps sustain your energy levels due to its satiating effect, which may help prevent your moods from fluctuating.

Whole-food carbohydrate sources: Carbohydrates come from foods such as grains, legumes, and fruits, and from sweeteners such as honey, sugar, and maple syrup. Carbohydrates break down into glucose, your brain's main source of energy. Your brain needs a steady supply of glucose. This ensures your body and brain function optimally and you have good energy levels. Carbohydrates also help reduce the stress hormone cortisol. The trick with carbohydrate-rich foods is to have foods with a low-glycemic load, that is, foods that will have less of a burden on your blood sugar levels. Also, eating carbohydrates with a source of protein, fat, and fiber—for example a meal that contains meat (or eggs etc.), rice, and vegetables—helps slow down the release of carbohydrates into your blood, making them much more energy sustaining and mood balancing.

Foods that are rich in B vitamins: B vitamins are very important for your nervous system, neurotransmitter production, blood health, and energy production. Your energy is produced in your cells' factory, the mitochondria. B vitamins are found in many different foods. B vitamins from B_1 to B_{12} come from a range of foods including green leafy vegetables, animal products, dairy products, seeds, legumes, organ and muscle meats, nutritional yeasts, eggs, and fruits.

Antioxidant-rich fruits and vegetables: Colorful fruits and vegetables are sources of many vitamins, minerals, antioxidants, and phytochemicals, all important for a healthy brain and body.

Essential fatty acid–rich foods: Your brain is largely made up of fat. One type of fat that is especially important for brain health is essential fatty acids. Essential fatty acids, best found in whole foods such as fish and seafood, are also anti-inflammatory, which is important for overall brain health. Essential fatty acids are needed for the health of your brain's neurons.

Water: Drinking sufficient water is important for perfusion, the blood flow to the brain. Water is also important for blood volume and keeping the body's temperature regulated. Try infusing water with certain spices to make teas for a calming and relaxing, as well as hydrating, experience.

Spice Actions for Brain and Mental Health

Spices that are particularly beneficial for brain and mental health include those with nervine, adaptogen, adrenal, anti-inflammatory, and antioxidant actions. The following list details how these help with mental health and brain function.

- **Nervine:** Nervine and nervine tonics are medicinal plants that act to support and relax the mind, and calm the nervous system. They also help strengthen and restore health to the nervous system.
- **Adaptogen:** An adaptogen helps you to adapt to stress and increases your resilience to stress.
- **Adrenal tonic:** An adrenal tonic is thought to "tone" your adrenal glands, support your nervous system, and increase your ability to cope with stress.
- **Anti-inflammatory:** An anti-inflammatory medicinal plant is one that reduces inflammation.
- **Antioxidant:** An antioxidant is something that can help inhibit oxidative stress.

Spices for Brain Health and Better Memory

Herbs and spices can be part of a preventative plan to keep the brain in a healthy condition. Your cognition can be positively influenced by your diet and by including certain foods and spices. Here are a few spices that may help improve your brain health:

- **Turmeric:** Turmeric (*Curcuma longa*) is thought to be useful for brain health due to its antioxidant properties. Western herbal medicine regards it as an "anti-Alzheimer's" herb.
- **Ginger:** Ginger (*Zingiber officinale*) is another spice for memory and cognitive function. Ginger is thought to be beneficial in improving cognition due to its ability to reduce oxidative stress. Ginger was tested in a double-blind, placebo-controlled randomized trial by Naritsara Saenghong and Jintanaporn Wattanathorn (2012). They wanted to determine the effect of an extract of ginger on cognitive ability and working memory in women. Sixty women were given either a placebo or capsular ginger extract (40 mg or 800 mg) once a day. The researchers found that ginger has potential as a cognitive-enhancing spice in postmenopausal women. Ginger also helps increase circulation and has anti-inflammatory properties.
- **Peppermint and pepper:** Peppermint and pepper are both circulatory stimulants. Peppermint is also a nervine, which helps relax and calm the nervous system. It is also suitable to help reduce tension and anxiety.
- **Rosemary:** Rosemary is an herb traditionally used to improve memory and retention of information. You can use rosemary simply by just putting a few drops

of essential oil on a tissue and smelling it while studying and learning. You can also add rosemary to an oil burner or even just smell a stem of rosemary leaves. A study published in the *Medical Journal of the Islamic Republic of Iran* in 2015 examined rosemary extract to see whether it affects spatial memory, learning, and antioxidant enzymes in the hippocampus. Middle-aged rats were given either 50 mg, 100 mg, or 200 mg of the rosemary extract. The researchers found that after twelve weeks the rats who had 100 mg per kilo of body weight of rosemary extract had an increased score of spatial memory and an increase in antioxidant enzymes. Rosemary can also be consumed as an infusion or taken as an herbal tincture, which your herbalist may prescribe. Rosemary is also great eaten on roasted vegetables or meats.

- **Cocoa:** Here's some good news for (dark) chocolate lovers! Cocoa may have some beneficial effects in reducing cognitive decline. A trial by Daniela Mastroiacovo et al. (2014) looked at the effect of cocoa flavonoids, a type of antioxidant, on cognitive performance in elderly people. This study was designed as a double-blind, controlled, and parallel-arm study. Ninety people who did not have any signs of cognitive dysfunction were examined every day for eight weeks. They were given a drink that contained 993 mg of cocoa flavonoids (high in flavonols), a drink with 520 mg (intermediate flavonols), or a drink that had 48 mg (low in flavonols). Their cognitive function was assessed at the start of the study and at the end. The authors concluded in the study that regular consumption of cocoa flavonoids "can reduce some measures of age-related cognitive dysfunction."

Spices for Less Stress and Happier Moods

Not only do herbs and spices help increase your mood with their vibrant colors, aromas, and tastes, but they can also have a physiological effect on your stress levels, moods, emotions, and anxieties. The popularity of natural medicines in treating mental health is increasing due to their effectiveness and minimal side effects, compared to some drug therapies. Of course, pharmacological drugs have their place so please assess with your doctor to see what is right for you. Spices can be used safely in the diet, within normal amounts.

In naturopathic medicine and herbal medicine, some spices (and many herbs) can help you improve your stress tolerance and reduce inflammation, whereas others help you relax and support your nervous system. Here are some examples:

Rose

Rose (*Rosa spp.*), from the Rosaceae family, is a great example of a spice that can have a positive effect on your emotional and mental health. Roses have long been used for their beauty, aroma, and therapeutic benefits.

Many fragrant varieties of rose can be used therapeutically. According to Youssef and Mousa's article in *Food and Public Health*, roses may have "antidepressant, antiviral, antibacterial and anti-inflammatory" actions.

Australian naturopath and herbalist Clara Bitcon says of rose that "any fragrant garden variety is perfect (just ensure they haven't been sprayed). Rose relaxes and opens the heart, and if taken over a period of time, can help us to heal and let go of past grief, sadness and hurt, and restores trust. Many healing traditions believe that a wounded or closed heart blocks energy to the creative centres below, physically and emotionally."

Bitcon goes on to say that "roses are cooling and cleansing to the blood, and are therefore used for a number of different health complaints where inflammation is an underlying factor. However it is its emotionally supportive qualities that are most relevant for modern women. Bring rose into your life whenever you're going through a period of emotional imbalance, which can include PMS, menopausal mood swings, or any such time in your life when the cards dealt are rocking your center."

Rose petals were investigated in a study by Miho Igarashi and Chorong Song in the *Journal of Alternative and Complementary Medicine* (2014). They looked at whether fresh rose flowers could have an effect on heart rate variability by olfactory stimulation (smelling). They found that rose petals "induced a significant increase in parasympathetic nervous activities and an increase in "comfortable" and "natural" feelings." So just smelling roses has a positive benefit!

Roses can also be used in other beneficial ways, including in cooking. American herbalist Kiva Rose uses roses in internal preparations for a variety of reasons including emotions such as trauma, panic, fear, and stress in children, adults, and animals. She describes rose as being "calming, pleasant, blood moving" and says that its "mild nervine" action makes it "calming without sedating." It is also antispasmodic, and can be used internally or externally for mild to moderate cramps. Kiva also explains that it is wonderful at "opening the heart and restoring emotional equilibrium."

Rose petals and rose hips, especially, are a rich source of vitamin C. Vitamin C is needed to recycle an endogenous antioxidant called glutathione. Glutathione is your body's main antioxidant. Vitamin C is also needed for the production of the adrenal hormones such as norepinephrine, and neurotransmitters such as serotonin, the "happy hormone."

Saffron

Saffron refers to the stigmas of the *Crocus sativus* plant. The petals can also be used as well as the stigmas. Saffron is most famous for its bright coloring, which is often used to make rice yellow in dishes such as paella. Saffron may have antidepressive actions. A meta-analysis study by Hausenblas and Saha (2013) looked at the anti-depressive effects of saffron. Based on the five clinical trials that were analyzed they found that there may be evidence to support the use of saffron in those with major depressive disorder. A study by researchers Hossein Hosseinzadeh and Hani M. Younesi (2002) looked at saffron for its potential use as an anti-nociceptive (pain-reducing), anti-inflammatory, and anti-oedematous agent. The constituents from saffron petals and stigmas were extracted by water and ethanol for use in the study. Mice were given an acetic acid solution to induce abdominal constrictions. The mice were then given the extracted saffron preparations to see whether there was an effect on inflammation, edema, and nociception. The petal extracts showed less anti-inflammatory action than the extracts of the stigma on inflammation in the mice. Edema was also found to be reduced in the mice. The authors of the study concluded that both the water and ethanol extracts of saffron petals and the stigma have properties that may act as antinociceptive agents and could have effects in acute or chronic inflammatory conditions.

Licorice

According to the *British Herbal Pharmacopoeia* (1983), licorice (*Glycyrrhiza glabra*) is an "adrenal agent." Licorice, or liquorice as it is sometimes called, is used in herbal medicine to help increase stress resistance, improve stress tolerance, and reduce inflammation. Licorice's therapeutic actions include being an adrenal tonic and an adaptogen. Licorice has these effects by its actions on mineralocorticoids in the body, as it is able to turn cortisol into its inactive form, which prolongs its action. Licorice is naturally sweet and is used traditionally in certain beverages such as sambuca (in essential oil form), candies, and in certain herbal tea mixes too. However, the use of licorice does come with risks, so licorice is best used under supervision of a qualified health practitioner.

Licorice can increase blood pressure when used improperly, as it affects sodium and potassium levels.

✅ Fact

Licorice root was originally used to flavor licorice confectionery products. These days licorice is much more likely to be flavored with aniseed or fennel, which have similar flavors, although not botanically related.

Green Tea, Dill, and Sage

Dill (*Anethum graveolens*) and sage (*Salvia officinalis*) are both thought to have a calming effect on the nervous system. Green tea leaves (*Camellia sinensis*) contain the constituent L-theanine. Green tea has a relaxing and anxiolytic effect on your central nervous system, helping you to stay alert and focused. It has been found to be effective in those who are highly anxious and stressed by modulating the resting state of the brain. Green tea helps to do this by L-theanine's action on glutamate receptors, which affect agitation. Green tea is thought to increase alpha activity in the brain.

Caution with Certain Spices and Mental Health Issues

When living with mental health issues it is always best to seek the help of a qualified practitioner. Licorice can affect blood pressure levels, even in a short time, so it should only be prescribed by a qualified herbalist or naturopath.

In normal use, nutmeg (*Myristica fragrans*) is considered a safe and a delicious ingredient in many kinds of dishes. Nutmeg is considered to be an aphrodisiac. While some herbs and spices can cause positive effects on the brain and nervous system, other spices may not be suitable. While nutmeg is a delicious garnish on custards and in eggnog, too much nutmeg can cause disastrous results. It can unfortunately cause hallucinations as well as gastrointestinal complaints. According to the International Programme on Chemical Safety, there are risks with nutmeg as it can cause "transient psychosis, transient renal toxicity, and there is the possibility of fatty liver and hepatic necrosis, it is possibly a carcinogen, teratogenic, and there is a possibility of death." Symptoms of nutmeg intoxication include profuse "sweating, a flushed face, delirium, hallucinations, and confusion." Additionally other symptoms of nutmeg poisoning have been reported to include vomiting, tachycardia, agitation, and nausea. The toxic effects of nutmeg are thought to be caused by its constituent called myristicin, which is part of its essential oil content. To avoid these effects only use nutmeg in small amounts such as a sprinkle.

CHAPTER 7

Spices for Muscle and Skeletal Health

Your musculoskeletal system consists of your skeleton, bones, muscles, joints, ligaments, and tendons. It is responsible for the movement and strength of your body. Keeping your musculoskeletal system in good shape is important for overall body health. If you find that you are having issues with skeletal or muscle pain, the heating and cooling natures of some spices and culinary herbs can be beneficial to improve musculoskeletal health. You can also adjust lifestyle and dietary measures to improve results as well.

Common Musculoskeletal Problems and Issues

Musculoskeletal problems are very common these days. According to the American Academy of Orthopaedic Surgeons, visits to physicians for musculoskeletal symptoms and complaints are in the millions and are often for knee, back, shoulder, and neck issues, among other complaints. Other common problems include arthritic conditions such as rheumatoid arthritis and osteoarthritis, back pain, osteoporosis, and delayed onset muscle soreness (DOMS), which can occur a few days after exercise.

What Affects Your Musculoskeletal System?

Sometimes, your lifestyle or dietary choices can adversely affect parts of your body without you even knowing it. This is true for your musculoskeletal system. The following issues can affect your musculoskeletal system if not corrected:

- **Immobility.** Immobility is a manifestation of the sedentary, busy lifestyles that are so common nowadays. But it doesn't have to be. You can work movement into your daily life and reduce the time you are sitting and immobile by taking breaks to stretch and move around, as well as incidental exercise, that is, physical activity that is part of your daily lifestyle such as hanging out washing or taking the stairs.
- **Over exercising.** A balance between a good amount of exercise and resting is important to avoid over straining the body and to allow the body to recover from exercise, repair itself, and build muscle.
- **Lack of weight-bearing exercises.** Weight-bearing exercises are essential for strength, muscle-building, and bone density.
- **Poor diet.** Diet can play an important role in strengthening the health of your bones and musculature.

Foods for Musculoskeletal Health and Wellness

What you eat may affect your musculoskeletal health. You may find that you are seeing improvement in your musculoskeletal health by eating a healthy diet and engaging in a good exercise and movement program.

Magnesium is a much favored mineral among nutritionists for its ability to help relax muscles and reduce muscular aches and tension. Magnesium is also important for energy production because of its function in the mitochondria (the energy factories in your cells), as a key nutrient in the citric acid cycle. Magnesium is found in many foods such as dark green leafy vegetables, including spinach, Swiss chard, and kale. It is also it is found in dark chocolate, nuts, seeds, and coffee.

 Alert

Essential fatty acids help reduce inflammation in your body. They are best consumed from whole foods such as fish and avocado and in smaller amounts of nuts and seeds.

Protein is an important macronutrient for building strong muscles and contributing to the strength of the bones. Protein comes from many foods such as meat including poultry, lamb, beef, seafood, and dairy foods, and also plant-based sources such as tofu and tempeh, beans, legumes, pulses, and nuts and seeds.

Spices for Musculoskeletal Health

Spices have many uses in keeping your muscles and skeletal system healthy. They can help with reducing inflammation and pain, increasing circulation and nutrients supply, and reducing excess fluid. They may be used topically for pain-relieving and anti-inflammatory purposes. Conditions that spices may be useful for are muscle pain (such as DOMS), arthritis, joint stiffness, muscular cramps and aches, and in assisting in recovery after exercise.

 Fact

Inflammation is one of the causes of pain in some musculoskeletal conditions. Though inflammation is protective, ongoing and chronic inflammation may be detrimental to the body and prevent healing.

Spices for Internal Use

Spices can be used internally, by consuming them as tea or with food in a meal in order to give your body therapeutic phytochemicals and nutrients. Spices can be taken to help improve joint health and muscle health by reducing pain and inflammation, which may improve joint stiffness and reduce muscular pain. Spices that can be used internally for these purposes include celery seed, ginger, turmeric, and rose hips.

- **Celery seed:** Celery seed is known to have a diuretic action. Diuretics help the body to increase diuresis (urination) and therefore the body can excrete excess fluid from the buildup of inflammation and edema. For example, if joints are inflamed, using celery seed may help reduce fluid buildup and secondarily help reduce pain associated with inflammation. This is partly why celery seed is used in gout. Celery seed is also a depurative spice, which means that it is traditionally used to improve the quality of the blood and acts as a blood cleanser. Celery seed can also help with reducing pain as well.

- **Ginger:** Ginger rhizome/root (*Zingiber officinale*) is an anti-inflammatory spice. Ginger is indicated for those who have poor circulation and feel cold often. It is a spice that is traditionally used and indicated for arthritis and joint pain. When taken internally as food or a tea, or in extract form, it can help reduce inflammation, which may be suitable for those with certain joint complaints and issues.

- **Turmeric:** Turmeric (*Curcuma longa*) is an anti-inflammatory spice that is useful for the musculoskeletal system. Turmeric and some of its constituents, including curcumin, have been well researched and proven effective for many inflammatory conditions, including arthritis.

- **Rose hips:** According to researcher Dr. Lesley Braun, rose hips from the *Rosa canina* (dog rose) plant may have anti-inflammatory and antinociceptive (pain-reducing) activity. Rose hips have been investigated in people with osteoarthritis and it was found that symptoms of pain were reduced. Rose hips are a natural source of vitamin C and flavonoids. Rose hips can be eaten in the form of a rose hip syrup, or in supplement form as prescribed by your healthcare practitioner.

Spices for Topical (External) Uses

Spices and other medicinal plants can be used topically to warm or cool certain areas such as sore muscles, and to provide pain relief, reduce inflammation, and increase blood flow.

- **Horseradish:** Horseradish contains the constituent glucosinolate. Glucosinolate is what gives horseradish its strong and pungent taste. Horseradish can be used in external preparations to help stimulate blood flow to a local area.
- **Mustard:** Mustard also contains glucosinolates and has similar actions to horseradish. Mustard is also warming and can increase circulation to the area which it is applied. It is anti-inflammatory as well. A mustard poultice can be used to help reduce muscle soreness and to warm muscles. A mustard poultice can be made by mixing crushed mustard seed into a paste with water, wrapping it up in a piece of cloth, and then using this as a compress on sore muscle, joints, or areas with irritated nerves. Avoid sensitive skin and areas that are dry, irritated, or have broken skin. Make sure to check the skin every few minutes to reduce chances of a burn, which may occur if left on too long.

- **Ginger:** Ginger is a very warming and anti-inflammatory spice. You can use ginger on sore muscles by cooking up a decoction of 4 cups of water and 1 small whole grated gingerroot. Leave it to cool and then you can dip a cloth in it and apply this cloth as a compress on sore muscles. This can bring a warming sensation to wherever it is applied and may help reduce pain. Make sure to check the skin and avoid leaving it on too long to avoid burns.
- **Chili:** The fruit and seeds of the chili (*Capsicum spp.*) plant can be used not only in cooking but also for external applications. Topically, cayenne can act as a rubefacient, as it a very warming spice. It can help increase blood circulation to whatever area it is applied. Cayenne contains the constituent capsaicin. According to the Mayo Clinic, capsaicin can be used to help relieve shingles and pain associated with muscular strains or rheumatoid arthritis. Capsaicin affects the nociceptors, reduces nerve pain, and acts as a local analgesic (pain-reducer).
- **Frankincense:** Frankincense is from the *Boswellia* species of plants. In herbal medicine, frankincense, a resin, is used to treat musculoskeletal conditions. It can be used topically, as an essential oil, or diluted in a carrier oil. M.Z. Siddiqui (2011) says that *Boswellia serrata*, which is used in Ayurveda, is beneficial for arthritis, is anti-inflammatory, and is an analgesic (pain-reliever).

Alert

Certain spices (and foods) may be cautioned in those with joint issues and those sensitive to plants from the Solanaceae, or nightshade, family. Plants from the Solanaceae family include tomatoes, potatoes, and chilies.

Beyond adding spices and nutrient-rich food to your diet, outside help is always recommended. The first point of call would be your general practitioner. Physical therapists and massage therapists can also help you assess and treat your issues and you may be referred to one by your doctor. Qualified naturopathic and nutritional medicine practitioners can be of assistance, too, to help develop tailored nutritional plans that help you reduce inflammation and pain.

CHAPTER 8

Spices for Beautiful Skin

Spices can be useful to include in food and in teas for specific skin disorders and also for general skin health. Certain spices can also be eaten or used on the skin topically for a healing and therapeutic effect. You can use spices in a range of ways to help improve the health of your skin and integumentary system. The skin is your largest organ by weight. It functions as a strong external covering as part of your immune system, to help protect against any infections or pathogens. It protects your body and also helps regulate your body temperature.

Skin Disorders

Skin conditions are a common occurrence and are all too familiar for many people these days. Skin conditions can take a while to resolve due to their complexity and because there can be many causes and triggers. Some of the most common skin conditions include acne, dandruff, eczema (dermatitis), rosacea, and psoriasis.

Acne

Acne is a skin condition characterized by blockage and eruption of the hair follicles and sebaceous follicles of the skin, which can result in cysts, blackheads, pustules, and papules. Acne can be inflammatory or noninflammatory and may have open or closed comedones. In inflammatory acne, when the inflammation is close to the skin, it causes pustules. And when inflammation is deeper in the skin, papules and cystic nodules form. Acne is thought to be exacerbated by the microbe *Propionibacterium acnes*, which infects the skin, though this bacterium is normally friendly. Acne is also thought to be affected by an imbalance of androgens, sex hormones, such as dihydrotestosterone, formed from testosterone. Other factors that affect acne include an imbalance of prostaglandins and inflammation, and excess sebum production. Some may find that certain dietary components worsen acne too.

Rosacea, Eczema, and Psoriasis

Rosacea is an inflammatory skin condition where blood vessels in the face have become enlarged, making the face appear red. Rosacea is also known as acne rosacea. The blood vessels in the skin can become enlarged due to vasodilation, and they can even become bulbous. The four sub types of rosacea are erythematotelangiectatic, papulopustular, phymatous, and ocular rosacea.

Eczema, also known as dermatitis, is an inflammatory condition of the skin. If you suffer from eczema you may notice your skin is itchy and red, and there might be pus as well. Eczema may be caused by allergens and infections, and can be associated with "atopic" conditions (such as asthma and hay fever), and anything that can irritate the skin such as chemicals. Different types of eczema include atopic dermatitis, diaper dermatitis, irritant contact dermatitis, and seborrheic dermatitis.

Dandruff is a type of eczema. Signs of dandruff include a dry scalp that is flaky and it may be itchy too. Dandruff is thought to be caused by yeasts called *Malassezia*, which are normally friendly on the scalp, but have become rogue.

Psoriasis is a condition where the skin develops proliferative, scaly plaques. Inflammation is involved in psoriasis and is affected by autoimmune processes. Subtypes of psoriasis include plaque psoriasis, guttate psoriasis, erythrodermic psoriasis, and pustular psoriasis.

Spice Actions for Beautiful Skin

For healthy skin you need good blood circulation to transfer the nutrients your body has digested around your body. Your skin can also benefit from traditional spices (and herbs) in your diet to aid in production and maintenance of skin health. Spices can help improve the overall function and structure of your skin by offering constituents and actions that are antimicrobial, antiandrogenic, anti-inflammatory, wound healing, liver tonics, peripheral circulatory stimulants, antioxidant-rich, and astringent.

Some herbs and spices can be used directly on your skin, such as those that are emollient, which soothe the skin; others have a secondary and systemic effect in your body to improve skin quality through improving blood circulation to tissues around the skin. By including these spices in your diet, you can reap their nutritional and medicinal benefits and you may be on your way to having healthier skin.

Circulatory Stimulants

Spices help heal and nourish the skin by increasing blood circulation to the peripheries and onward to the skin. If you want healthy, vibrant skin you need good blood circulation to help transfer nutrients to where they need to go. Spices that can help improve circulation are generally very warming to taste and in their action. They are termed circulatory or peripheral circulation stimulants. These include ginger, chili, and black pepper.

 Fact

Did you know that there is a connection between your gastrointestinal tract and your skin? Your gut health can reflect your skin health and vice versa. This is part of a connection called the gut–skin axis.

Hepatics and Liver Detoxifiers

The liver can impact the health of your skin and is very important for good skin condition, as well as overall body health. You can assist your liver to help transform the nutrients you eat into forms your body can use effectively, as well as enhance your liver's detoxification process. Having a healthy liver is important for reducing excess hormones in skin conditions such as dihydrotestosterone (DHT), as part of the acne presentation, and estrogen.

Antiandrogenics and Antimicrobials

Some spices may help the body balance certain sex hormones, called androgens, reduce excess testosterone in the form of dihydrotestosterone (DHT), and reduce excess sebum production and inflammation, which exacerbates acne. Antimicrobial spices help the body to combat bacterial infections and reduce infections in the skin and the body.

Anti-Inflammatories, Diaphoretics, and Emollients

Many spices are anti-inflammatory and they may assist in reducing inflammation in the skin as well as pain, excess sebum production, and sores.

Some "hot" tasting spices help the body to increase sweating or diaphoresis, which is the technical term for sweating. Sweating is important for skin health as it helps the skin to mobilize lymphatic fluid.

Emollient plants are those that soothe skin (topically) and are mucilaginous due to mucopolysaccharides. These herbs and spices can help reduce inflammation topically. They may also be suitable to apply on ulcerations, burns, scalds, and rashes.

Foods for Beautiful Skin

In order for your skin to be strong and beautiful it needs to be fed the right nutrients. A nutritious diet helps to provide your body with the building blocks for strong, beautiful skin.

When you eat a nutritious diet you are helping to provide your body with the nutrients and cofactors for healthy skin.

Animal Proteins, Meat, and Eggs

Animal proteins such as beef, poultry, and seafood are an important source of protein, zinc, iron, and B vitamins. Protein and zinc are especially beneficial and necessary for strong, healthy skin. Protein is a macronutrient, which is important for the repair and renewal of your skin. Protein-rich foods include beef, eggs, dairy products, seafood, and legumes. Zinc is important for wound healing and the immune system and is found in foods such as red meat, oysters, seafood, and pumpkin seeds. Eggs are a source of lecithin, which is helpful for the digestion and emulsion of fats, as well as being a source of protein.

Fish, Nuts, and Seeds

Fish, nuts, and seeds are sources of essential fatty acids. Fish and seafood are sources of essential fatty acids (EFAs) in forms that are much easier for the body to use, while nuts and seeds have pre-formed versions, which your body has to convert, and are not always as efficiently converted.

You may be deficient in EFAs if you find you have dry skin, hair, nails, and eyes. You can eat EFAs in many foods such as fish, nuts, seeds, avocado, flaxseed and oil, and other cold-pressed oils.

Vitamin A–Rich Foods

Vitamin A is a fat-soluble vitamin found in many foods from animal products including butter, ghee, cheese, and other dairy products, and also in liver and seafood. The group of pre-formed versions of vitamin A, called carotenoids, can be found in plant foods, such as carrots, spinach and other dark green leafy vegetables, as well as pumpkin and sweet potato. In the skin and in the body, vitamin A is needed for cell differentiation, growth, and gene expression. Vitamin A is also important for immune system health.

Colorful Fruits and Vegetables

Colorful fruits and vegetables offer many benefits and therapeutic properties to the body and the health of the skin. Vitamin C is found in many foods including fresh fruits such as berries and colorful, bright vegetables. Berries are also a source of anthocyanins, the blue, red, and purple pigments in berries and other plant foods that are a type of phytochemicals called flavonoids. Antioxidants are protective to the fats in the cell membranes and in the skin. Beta-carotene is an orange pigment in plants such as carrots and pumpkin. Lycopene, a red pigment, is found naturally in foods such as cooked tomatoes.

Water and Water-Rich Foods

Water is needed for hydrating the cells and keeping the skin "plump" and healthy. Water is needed for adequate blood supply around the body, to support skin health. Water is also needed for the flow of lymphatic fluid, important for removal of wastes in the body. You can drink water as it is, and in herbal teas and drinks. You can also get some water from food such as soups, and many types of vegetables and fruits including cucumbers, aloe vera, carrots, pineapple, and watermelon. You can also get some water from fresh juices. You may like to add spices to some juices. Go ahead and add spices such as a bit of cayenne pepper or turmeric for flavor and their therapeutic benefits.

Bitter and Sour Foods

Bitter foods, such as dandelion, dark chocolate, coffee, and bitter greens, stimulate your gut to help your digestive system function well. Sour foods such as lemon juice, lime juice, apple cider vinegar, and raw sauerkraut have similar actions to bitter foods too, though they may be contraindicated in conditions such as GERD. A strong digestive system is critical for healthy skin, in order to extract all the nutrients in your food, and to support the health of your body.

Spices for Beautiful, Healthy Skin

Certain spices and herbs that may help skin health include circulatory stimulants, those that improve skin function, antiandrogenics, antimicrobials, and those with anti-inflammatory, diaphoretic, and emollient actions.

Turmeric

Turmeric (*Curcuma longa*) can be used topically as well as internally as an ingredient in food and drinks. Turmeric is indicated in inflammatory and bacterial conditions of the skin due to its anti-inflammatory and antibacterial actions. Turmeric can also be used as an inflammation-reducing face mask, though it can stain the skin. Turmeric, in the form of oil, has been shown to have antifungal properties against a type of fungi called dermatophytes (tinea, or ringworm) according to authors Mukda Jankasem and Mansuang Wuthi-udomlert (2013).

Rosemary

Rosemary (*Rosmarinus officinalis*) is used often as a therapeutic plant in herbal medicine, and of course as an herb in cooking. Rosemary is an antioxidant-rich herb. It is also a rubefacient, which is a topical irritant that helps increase circulation where it is applied on the skin. Rosemary is also anti-inflammatory, antibacterial, and a circulatory stimulant. Rosemary is another favorite of Mrs. Beeton. In her 1861 *Mrs. Beeton's Book of Household Management*, she recommended it as an herb to "promote the growth of hair." She suggested olive oil, spirit of rosemary, and a few drops of nutmeg to be mixed together and applied to the roots of the hair to help stimulate hair growth. Rosemary is thought to help stimulate blood flow to the brain and scalp and is often used to stimulate hair growth today. Rosemary essential oil can be added to shampoo or conditioner. It can also be made into a strong infusion and used as a hair wash. Rosemary is also thought to aid in detoxification of the liver. Rosemary is an aromatic bitter herb, which may help stimulate digestive secretions, thus improving digestive function.

Rose Petal and Rose Hip

Quite a few parts of roses can be used in skin conditions. The rose hips, from the buds of roses, are often made into an oil and can be used topically on the skin to soothe and nourish the skin. Rose hips can also be cooked to be made into a syrup with sugar or honey and can be eaten. Rose hips are a rich source of vitamin C, antioxidants, and flavonoids. Of these nutrients, vitamin C is especially important as it is an antioxidant and is needed to help produce collagen in the skin. Rose petals have also been studied in regard to their antimicrobial actions on the skin. Rose petals are astringent and anti-inflammatory, and are thought to aid in wound healing. Rose water can be used on the skin as a toner due to its astringent action and beautiful aroma, which also makes it useful as a natural perfume. You can use rose petals in a face scrub with a bit of sugar to gently exfoliate your face as well.

Cinnamon

Cinnamon contains mucilage, which can be used to reduce inflammation and soreness on the skin. Cinnamon is also antibacterial, so it may be good for skin conditions of a bacterial nature. You can make a face mask with a bit of powdered cinnamon, manuka honey, and uncooked and ground rolled oats and gently scrub this mixture on your skin. After application, wash this off your face and moisturize as per your normal routine.

Myrrh

Myrrh can be used as a topical treatment for acne. Myrrh is anti-inflammatory, supports wound healing, and is astringent and antibacterial, so it can be beneficial for improving certain skin conditions such as acne.

Licorice

In acne, there can be a hormonal aspect where androgens are imbalanced. Licorice may help balance androgens and testosterone, so may be suitable for hormonal acne, including acne presented in women with polycystic ovarian syndrome (PCOS). Licorice is also soothing and emollient on the skin due to its mucilaginous properties.

Peppermint and Green Tea

Peppermint and green tea are both plants that can be used as refreshing teas. They are also both plants that may help reduce excess androgens in acne. Peppermint is also particularly cooling, refreshing, and anti-inflammatory. Green tea is rich in antioxidants, which are protective to skin cells and beneficial for skin health. Cooled peppermint tea can also act as a soothing toner for your skin, especially in summer. You can dab it on with cotton cloth.

Calendula

Calendula flowers are traditionally used for their anti-inflammatory and wound-healing properties. It is also a great flower to help stimulate lymphatic flow in the body, due to its lymphatic actions. Calendula is antibacterial and can be used topically as a face wash, in a scrub, or in a salve. It can also be consumed in a tea or in salads.

CHAPTER 9

Spices for a Healthy Cardiovascular System

Your cardiovascular system's anatomy includes the heart, arteries, blood vessels, capillaries, microvasculature, and the connections between them. Your cardiovascular system is very important as it transfers blood, nutrients, and oxygen around the body and helps transfer wastes out of the body. It is also important for its role in helping to regulate your body through the transfer of immune cells and hormones. It gets oxygen from the lungs and it can then take it around the body back up to your heart.

Cardiovascular Issues

Cardiovascular disease is a frequent occurrence in this modern age. There are certain factors that can contribute to a decline in cardiovascular function and health. Risk factors include smoking, high blood pressure, abnormal serum lipids, poor body composition and obesity, a diet high in processed foods, alcohol intake, and little to no exercise. You can prevent, change, or improve many of these risk factors through diet and lifestyle changes, but there are other risk factors we can't change. These include a family history of cardiovascular disease, your sex, your age, and (to a certain extent) your mental health. You can generally improve your cardiovascular health by avoiding *modifiable* risk factors. This is a part of preventive healthcare.

Causes of Cardiovascular Disease

There are many factors that are thought to contribute to the pathogenesis of cardiovascular disease. Some of these causes and contributing issues include atherosclerosis, inflammation, oxidative stress, poor diet, and obesity.

Atherosclerosis

Coronary artery atherosclerosis is the main cause of cardiovascular disease. In coronary artery atherosclerosis, the walls of the coronary arteries become damaged due to fat deposits in the inner artery walls. The mechanisms involved in atherosclerosis include endothelial damage, which oxidizes the cholesterol and causes accumulation in the arterial walls. Specific types of white blood cells that have turned into macrophages cause lipids to accumulate and form part of the atherosclerosis.

Inflammation

Inflammation is thought to be a key driver in the development of cardiovascular issues and disease. In *Frontiers in Physiology* in 2014, the authors state: "We currently believe that atherosclerosis is an inflammatory disease." Your risk of heart disease and inflammation can be tested by your doctor. Herbs, spices, diet, sleep, and exercise can all play a role in reducing and modulating inflammation.

Oxidative Stress

Put simply, an oxidant is something that causes damage in the body, and an antioxidant helps reduce it. Oxidative stress is the result of free-radical damage. Oxidation happens in the plant world too. Have you ever taken a bite of an apple and then a while later the section where you have bitten has turned brown? That is oxidation at work. Oxidation is the chemical process in which there is a gain of electrons by free radicals that are free to attach to cells, which subsequently damages the cells. Oxidation happens to metals, such as tin, as well. The rusting of metals is an example of oxidation. Oxidative stress in the human body can be thought of similarly. Antioxidants help your body to counteract oxidation. You can get antioxidants from your diet, but your body also makes its own strong antioxidants quite effectively. Oxidation is thought to affect cholesterol too.

Poor Diet and Obesity

What you eat can affect the health of your cardiovascular system. It is well known that a processed, refined, and hyper caloric diet (in the absence of exercise) can contribute to obesity and the breakdown of your cardiovascular system. Specifically, steer clear of diets high in sugar, alcohol, and poor-quality fats, and low in nutrient-rich food. Having a high amount of body fat can put you at greater risk for cardiovascular issues including high blood pressure and high cholesterol, as well as metabolic dysfunction issues. According to the journal *Circulation* (2006), obesity is associated with conditions such as cardiovascular disease, type 2 diabetes, certain cancers, and sleep apnea.

Actions for the Cardiovascular System

Foods, herbs, and spices have many actions that are beneficial for the health of your cardiovascular system. Herbs, spices, and foods that may promote a healthy cardiovascular system have anti-inflammatory, antioxidant, circulatory stimulant, blood pressure, and cholesterol-lowering agents.

- **Anti-Inflammatory:** Anti-inflammatory spices are indicated for the health of this system due to their ability to systemically reduce inflammation around the body. This is especially important in cardiovascular health as there can be inflammation as a part of certain cardiovascular conditions.

- **Circulatory Stimulant:** Circulatory stimulants help increase the peripheral circulation in the body, which may be beneficial for those with cold hands and feet and poor circulation.
- **Blood Pressure Lowering:** Particular medicinal plants can have a beneficial effect on the cardiovascular system by helping to decrease blood pressure.
- **Cholesterol Lowering:** Certain medicinal plants, and some spices, may have a cholesterol-lowering effect or may help the body to support cholesterol management.
- **Antispasmodic:** Spices that possess antispasmodic properties may help relax muscles and potentially relax blood vessels, which may help in reducing blood pressure.
- **Mucilaginous:** Mucilaginous and fiber-rich foods and spices may have a beneficial effect on the cardiovascular system and health.

Alert

An antioxidant is something that helps to quench free radicals, reducing oxidative stress and damage.

Tips for a Healthy Cardiovascular System

Looking after your cardiovascular system requires a holistic and preventative approach. A good dose of regular exercise, stress reduction, avoiding smoking, and adequate sleep are as important as including foods that are fiber-rich in the diet such as oats (which contain beta-glucan), apples, phylum husk, and other sources of soluble fiber that help reduce cholesterol.

The following are some general tips to promote cardiovascular health:

- **Antioxidant-Rich Foods:** Antioxidant-rich foods help support the general health of the cardiovascular system and reduce oxidative stress. Antioxidants come from a variety of foods such as brightly colored fruits and vegetables such as berries and tomatoes (as a source of lycopene), as well as nuts and seeds.
- **Salt Intake:** Excess salt intake is generally thought to be detrimental for the cardiovascular system, especially in those who have high blood pressure. Excess salt is mainly found in processed foods.
- **Fiber-Rich Foods:** Fiber can be found in a range of fruits, vegetables, nuts, seeds, grains (such as oats), and legumes and other plant fibers such as psyllium husk. Fiber-rich foods may help reduce blood cholesterol. They are thought to reduce cholesterol as they bind to bile in the gastrointestinal tract.
- **Fish, Nuts, and Seeds:** Fish, nuts, and seeds are a source of essential fatty acids (EFAs). EFAs are anti-inflammatory. Essential fatty acids may be beneficial in lowering cholesterol and blood pressure levels, too. However, in some people, fish oil may be contraindicated for those using certain heart medications, so always check with your doctor before supplementing. EFAs are better consumed in whole-food form such as in fish, rather than through capsules of fish oil, due to how readily fish oil can oxidize. As a whole food, fish is rich in protein as well as essential fatty acids.
- **B Vitamin–Rich Foods:** B vitamins, especially B_{12}, B_6, and B_9, are important to help the body reduce an inflammatory chemical called homocysteine. These B vitamins

can be found in foods such as animal proteins (B_{12}), green leafy vegetables, cereals, and fruits (B_6 and B_9).

- **Exercise:** Exercise cannot be underestimated for the benefits it gives your body as a whole and for the health of your cardiovascular system. Exercise helps improve lipoprotein and cholesterol levels and helps increase insulin sensitivity. It also helps improve body composition and reduces fat cell size.
- **Relaxation and Stress Reduction:** Getting enough sleep and adequate relaxation is important for whole-body health, as is reducing stress. Researchers Robert Schneider and Clarence Grim concluded in a 2012 trial that stress reduction has been associated with lower blood pressure and less psychosocial stress factors, and may be useful as secondary prevention of cardiovascular disease.
- **Managing Your Body Weight:** A healthy body weight is favorable for a healthy cardiovascular system, as is reducing obesity. Rena Wing and Wei Lang (2011) explain in *Diabetes Care* that even a 5–10 percent reduction of body weight can improve cardiovascular disease risk factors (such as better glycemic control, blood pressure, "good cholesterol," and triglycerides) in a time period of one year and great weight loss had even more associated benefits.

Spices for Cardiovascular Health

The foods you eat can be inflammatory and low in nutrients or your diet can be nutrient-rich, anti-inflammatory, and protective to your blood vessels and general heart health and cardiovascular system. Good food choices can be high in antioxidant properties too. Adding spices to your diet and lifestyle can make your diet super charged with nutrients that improve your cardiovascular health for the long term. Spices can also be effective to help increase peripheral circulation in the body, important for the transfer of nutrients around your body.

 Alert

Licorice (*Glycyrrhiza glabra*) is contraindicated in those with high blood pressure and any cardiovascular symptoms. Licorice can have this negative reaction even within a short time, such as a two-week period. Even licorice-flavored chewing gum may raise blood pressure in some people, so it is best to speak to your doctor.

How Spices Help Cardiovascular Health

Adding spices to your diet is one way to get additional nutrients that act in protective, anti-inflammatory, and nutrient-rich ways. Spices may also help improve cholesterol levels, increase antioxidant status, decrease blood pressure, and improve your cardiovascular system as a whole.

Garlic

Garlic (*Allium sativum*) may have some benefit in helping those with uncontrolled high blood pressure (hypertension) and for those with high cholesterol levels. Garlic's blood pressure lowering effects may be due to its ability to relax the blood vessels after vasodilation. According to researchers Karin Ried and Peter Fakler (2014), aged garlic extract was shown to increase thiol antioxidants including cysteine and glutathione (GSH) and reduce oxidative stress. GSH is one of your body's main endogenous (self-made) antioxidants. It is thought that garlic may have a positive benefit to help reduce blood pressure by certain mechanisms as explained by Karin Ried and Peter Fakler, which affect cysteine and GSH.

Cysteine and GSH affect nitric oxide production in the body, which in a series of reactions leads to smooth-muscle relaxation and lowered blood pressure. Garlic may have a positive effect on cholesterol levels, too.

According to Australian nutritionist Amanda Henham, garlic "is renowned these days for its use as an anti-platelet, cardiovascular (arterial health, blood pressure, high cholesterol), anti-bacterial and anti-viral, anti-inflammatory, and cancer prevention food. Many compounds and health promoting nutrients are found in garlic, creating a whole food with multiple benefits." She goes on to say, "When using garlic in cooking, it is a great idea to crush a clove or two and let it rest at room temperature to activate the enzymes required to increase the healing compounds. Add it as a last ingredient to numerous meals such as stir-fry, soups, casseroles, and sauces, and gently warm it. The active constituents may be lost from anything more than warming."

Whether garlic can reduce blood pressure and cholesterol levels is determined by diet and genetic responses. It is highly individualized and it is always best to talk to your doctor before changing your diet.

Hawthorn Berry and Rose

Hawthorn berry (*Crataegus oxyacantha*) is thought to be more of an herb than a spice, but it is worth mentioning due to how it can be used in cooking and because of its importance in the cardiovascular system. It is considered one of the best medicinal plants for protecting the heart and improving the health of the cardiovascular system. In the practice of herbal medicine, hawthorn berry is thought to be a hypotensive (blood-pressure lowering) and a cardiac tonic. Hawthorn berry is best used long term as it takes a while to work in the body. Hawthorn is rich in antioxidants called flavonoids. Hawthorn berry is botanically related to roses, both belonging to the Rosaceae family. Roses are thought to help the heart on an emotional level. Rose hips are a source of vitamin C, important for blood vessel health.

Roselle

The dark red petals of *Hibiscus sabdariffa* are rich in antioxidants, in the calyxes of the plant, called anthocyanins. These vibrant petals can be used to make a delicious red tea. Roselle is thought to be a great remedy to aid in reducing blood pressure due to its antioxidant content. Although, some meta-analyses have not always found consistent results that roselle lowers blood pressure. Because of the effect hibiscus has on lowering blood pressure, it is contraindicated in those with low blood pressure.

Green Tea

Green tea (*Camellia sinensis*) is thought to have beneficial effects on the central nervous system and it may also help relax the blood vessels. Green tea is a rich source of antioxidants called flavonoids. Some of green tea's main antioxidants are called catechins and they are protective to general cardiovascular health. According to a meta-analysis published in *Nature* in 2014, green tea may have a favorable and "significant" effect on decreasing blood pressure. Other studies have shown that green tea may be beneficial for lowering low-density lipoprotein cholesterol, as well as total cholesterol.

Turmeric

Turmeric (*Curcuma longa*) contains the constituent curcumin, which is a polyphenol. Turmeric and its constituents are rich in antioxidants and are anti-inflammatory. According to the *International Journal of Cardiology*, curcumin has been shown to be anti-inflammatory, antioxidant-rich, antithrombotic, anticarcinogenic, and protective to the cardiovascular system.

Wild Celery Seed and Cumin

Wild celery seed (*Apium graveolens*) may be useful in cardio-vascular health due to its potential as a diuretic, which increases urination and helps relieve retention of fluid. Celery seed is often used for its diuretic actions in conditions such as gout and rheumatism.

The common spice cumin (*Cuminum cyminum*), often used in curries, contains the antioxidants lutein and zeaxanthin. These carotenoid antioxidants are important for the health of micro-blood vessels, such as those in the eyes, and as such are beneficial for eye health.

Chili and Ginger

For those who generally have cold hands and feet, ginger may help with increasing your peripheral circulation. Ginger is energetically thought to be warming, as well as having a "spicy" and pungent taste. Chili is one of the strongest circulatory stimulants and "hot" spices. Only small amount of chili is needed to stimulate the peripheral circulation in the body and it is very effective in warming the body. The "hotness" of chili is measured by the Scoville scale.

Chili and ginger can be used together in meals or in a ginger tea (with a small pinch of fresh or dried chili).

 Fact

Cayenne is a great spice to use when it is snowing or if you are in the snow. You can use it by adding a little bit of powdered cayenne to your socks to keep your feet warm.

CHAPTER 10

Spices for Weight Loss

Spices can help complement your diet by increasing nutritional content and supporting weight loss. It can help to do this by supporting healthy blood sugar levels, increasing antioxidant status, and decreasing inflammation. Keep in mind that supporting and nourishing the body can put you on a good path for weight loss, as your body is getting the nutrients it needs to help support a healthy and well-balanced metabolism.

Obesity and the Modern Lifestyle

The current obesity problem found in many countries has just as much to do with diets as it does with lifestyles. Often, a sedentary lifestyle that lacks any consistent exercise can lead to weight gain. More so, poor diet and overeating can contribute to obesity as well.

Factors in Obesity

There are many factors that are involved in and contribute to the development of obesity. The following list details some of these factors:

- Dietary factors such as dietary excess and poor nutrient status and nutritional deficiencies
- Genetic factors
- Hormonal issues and conditions
- The gut microbiota and dysbiosis

- Excess inflammation
- Immobility, low to no exercise, and poor movement
- Stress
- Poor sleep or little sleep

"Diabesity" and Obesity

According to the European Commission the term *diabesity* was coined by scientist Eleazar Shafrir. Diabesity is the common presentation and association between obesity and diabetes, which are often seen together. In the journal *Obesity and Diabetes* (2013), Pilar Riobó Serván states that "there is a direct correlation between body mass index (BMI) and diabetes." There is also an inflammatory link between metabolic syndrome and obesity.

Obesity can make you immobile, it can lead to increased pressure on your joints, and it is pro-inflammatory. Obesity is also a risk factor for type 2 diabetes, hypertension, insulin resistance, cancer, atherosclerosis, and cardiovascular events. Conversely, losing fat and reducing obesity has many benefits associated with it, including prevention of many of the issues mentioned, as well as having a healthier, happier body.

Foods and Tips for Fat Loss

The context of your whole diet, rather than just individual components of your diet, is important when trying to lose weight. Fat loss takes time and it is better if it is slow, as a slower approach is more sustainable in the long run. Weight loss is better if your attitude is to adopt a long-term nutritious diet, rather than adopting a temporary fix-it-all diet. This will help you to see that eating can help make you healthier and it can help you to change your eating habits for good.

How to Improve Fat Loss

There are many factors that can definitely influence and decrease obesity, improve body composition, and improve weight loss. To lose weight certain things need to be taken into account. These things do include diet—what you're eating, when you're eating, and how often. Diet is important of course, but addressing your behaviors around food and your eating habits are more important. This is because behaviors are what can drive you to eat a certain way. Beyond your diet (i.e., the food you eat) you also need to consider exercise levels, stress, how well you are sleeping, your work-life balance, your emotions, and mental health, along with addressing any other underlying pathological cause.

Dietary Adjustments for Weight Loss

Here are some general guidelines for weight loss. It's important to identify any areas in your diet that are excesses (and deficiencies), which can affect your body's ability to lose fat and keep it off.

- Avoid sugar-sweetened beverages
- Don't fear fat
- Eat filling whole foods
- Eat your vegetables
- Eat protein-rich foods
- Drink water
- Avoid "diet" products
- Be mindful

These points are expanded in further detail in the following sections.

Avoid Sugar-Sweetened Beverages

Certain foods are very easy to over consume (and can contribute to weight gain). This is because they are highly refined and rich in calories but low in nutrients, protein, healthy fats, and fiber. These foods include soft drinks, candies, cakes, biscuits, fries, and other "snack" foods. Sometimes these foods and drinks are over-sweetened and use sugarcane or high-fructose corn syrup as a sweetener. Beverages contribute to weight gain as they are easy to drink and you may not realize how much sugar you have consumed by drinking them. When over consumed, they can contribute to fat gain.

Fact

Historically, sugar was actually used as a spice in small, medicinal quantities. This is much different from the 33 grams of sugar in each can of Coke.

Don't Fear Fat

Good, healthy fat can add valuable fat-soluble nutrients to your diet. Fats can also help keep you full and reduce your hunger. What are good, healthy fats? You can find healthy fats in a range of natural whole foods such as avocado, coconut, olives, nuts and seeds, fish and other seafood, eggs, beef, poultry, and pork. Specific healthy fats can come from a range of whole foods. Fish and seafood are a good source for essential fatty acids, the fats that help reduce inflammation and are important for brain health; avocados, olives, and olive oil contain monounsaturated fats; coconut oil is rich in medium-chain fatty acids; and whole animal products contain saturated fats, which are healthy in small amounts, as they provide energy for the body, as well as help you to feel satiated. Saturated fats are in foods such as unprocessed meats, butter, ghee, and eggs.

Alert

Many foods that are rich in saturated fat also contain other fats such as monounsaturated fats, as in the case of poultry, which are valuable for health and weight-loss.

The following list includes examples of foods and lifestyle choices that may assist with weight loss and overall health:

- **Eat Filling Whole Foods:** Your body needs certain nutrients to satisfy your appetite and keep you full, as well as healthy. These nutrients are best taken from whole, real foods.
- **Protein-Rich Foods:** Protein-rich foods help to keep you full and will help reduce cravings for other foods as you will be satiated.
- **Fiber-Rich Foods:** Some filling foods include those that contain soluble fiber such as oats, cooked root vegetables such as potatoes and sweet potato, and psyllium husk.
- **Vegetables:** Vegetables should be included as a part of your diet whether or not you want to lose weight. They can be a source of filling fiber, are good for your microbiome as they act as food ("prebiotics") for your gut bacteria, and of course they are very nutritious. They can be cooked in a variety of delicious ways, especially with the help of herbs and spices.
- **Water:** Water is very important for overall health. Adequate hydration also keeps you feeling full.
- **Avoid "Diet" Products:** Many products are marketed as "diet"; however, they are not products that support health or improve weight loss. Often they can be low in fat but are actually high in sugar and are not always health promoting, despite what the label might say.
- **Be Mindful about Food:** Being mindful means thinking about how, when, and what you eat. When you eat mindfully, you are not eating on the run, you take time to eat (when possible), and you enjoy your food. You are taking time to be conscious of what you are eating and not overindulging, just eating the right amount for

your hunger levels and to satiate you and fuel your body. Being mindful may help you lose weight as you are more conscious of what you put in your body.

- **Incorporate Exercise and Movement Into Your Day:** You can incorporate exercise by including incidental exercise, which helps you get movement in throughout your day, as well as more formal exercise throughout your week.

Spices for Weight Loss

Herbs and spices can complement a weight-loss program by adding flavor and nutritional and therapeutic benefits. Spices may offer benefits by enhancing weight loss and improving body composition and may affect certain markers for health. Spices can also be a lovely addition to a simple dish of steamed vegetables. They can be used to bring a great deal of flavor to a very basic dish.

Cinnamon

Cinnamon is an herb that is traditionally known for its sweet taste and also for helping to balance blood sugar levels. Australian naturopath Kelli Benjamin explains the benefits of cinnamon, saying, "If I had to choose one spice it would be cinnamon. It has the ability to delight the senses whilst quietly doing a world of good inside you—promoting healthy digestion and circulation, balancing blood sugar levels, reducing inflammation and preventing dementia. What more could you ask for? I had one client who had spent years on a roller-coaster of weight gain and depressive feelings due to her inability to manage sweet-cravings. She was resigned to having a sugar 'addiction.' I suggested she try cinnamon. Within a few days she emailed me the following: 'Thank you so much for suggesting the 1 teaspoon of cinnamon a day. I've started doing this and I haven't had any desire for sugar, which is incredible, considering what I have been experiencing on a daily basis. It's amazing.'"

Cinnamon can made into an herbal tea. You can add ½–¾ teaspoon of cinnamon powder to a cup of hot water. You can drink this up to three times a day, along with your meals.

Fenugreek

The seeds and green leafy parts of fenugreek (*Trigonella foenum-graecum*), or *methi* as it is known in Hindi, can be eaten in the diet. The seeds are what we use as a spice. The seeds are a source of soluble fiber and are thought to be a beneficial adjunct therapy for balancing blood sugar levels, as they have been traditionally used. A study in the *Journal of Nutrition and Metabolism* (2014) looked at obese and overweight individuals and the effect fenugreek has on postprandial blood sugar response, that is, the blood sugar response after meals. Although a small study, the individuals who were treated with fenugreek had a decreased postprandial response and an increased feeling of satiety (fullness).

Nigella

Nigella seed, botanically called *Nigella sativa*, is also known as black cumin seed. Nigella has been looked at in a few studies and its possible effects on those with metabolic syndrome has been investigated. In one study by Ramlah Mohamad Ibrahim and Nurul Syima Hamdan in 2014, nigella was examined to determine whether it has metabolic potential in women who are menopausal. While there wasn't a large effect on body composition, the researchers did find that nigella was protective by improving total cholesterol, triglycerides, low-density lipoprotein cholesterol, high-density lipoprotein cholesterol, and blood glucose in menopausal women. Another study by Latiffah Abdul Latiff and Saadat Parhizkar, also in 2014, researched how nigella would affect reproductive health and metabolic profiles in women who are perimenopausal. The women in the study were treated for twelve weeks with nigella. The treatment groups were shown to have a significant improvement in blood glucose and low-density lipoprotein cholesterol levels, as well as a reduction of the severity of some menopausal symptoms.

Green Tea

Traditionally green tea is believed to be associated with longevity and wellness. Green tea, *Camellia sinensis*, is also thought to be beneficial in weight loss. This could possibly be due to the antioxidants it contains, along with its caffeine content. According to the *Canadian Pharmacists Journal* (2014), green tea, in supplement form, has been shown to have some effects on weight loss. A meta-analysis by the *International Journal of Obesity* (2009) looked at the effects of green tea on weight loss and maintenance. They found that a type of antioxidant, called epigallocatechin gallate, and caffeine found in green tea had a positive effect on weight loss and weight management.

Chili

Chili plants, from the *Capsicum* genus, have long been believed to have "metabolism boosting" properties. Chili peppers contain capsaicinoids, which are thought to have bioactive properties. In a placebo-controlled, double-blind, randomized study in 2008, researchers Snitker and Fujishima looked at the effect of capsinoids on "fatness and energy metabolism in humans." The researchers found that the treatment group of subjects who were given oral capsinoids had a decrease in abdominal adiposity compared to the placebo group and that there was an increase in fat oxidation. A study by Josse and Sherriffs (2010) investigated how the consumption of capsinoids affects energy expenditure in humans. They mentioned that capsinoids are thermogenic (heat inducing) and promote fat oxidation.

CHAPTER 11

Additional Information and Spice *Materia Medica*

This spice *materia medica* details how certain spices (and some herbs) can be used therapeutically in food as part of a food-as-medicine approach. It includes monographs of some of the spices, and some herbs, used in this book. A monograph is an outline of an herb or spice that details information such as botanical name, common name, plant part, uses, and contraindications and cautions.

Spice Combinations, Cooking Ideas, and Uses

Spices can be combined with and complement a number of foods, drinks, and condiments. They can be used to flavor foods, which could be rather bland-tasting otherwise. Spices pair well in both sweet and savory dishes and have multipurpose uses. Herbs and spices, fruits, vegetables, grains, nuts, seeds, dairy, and animal products are often mixed together, in thousands of combinations.

Cautions and Contraindications

Generally, taking herbs and spices in the diet is okay within normal culinary amounts; however, if you're looking at therapeutic doses, you need to talk to your doctor. Having an increased amount above culinary amounts of certain spices may be contraindicated for some people, those on medication, those with high blood pressure, and in women who are pregnant or breastfeeding. If you are unsure, please speak to your doctor. Please note this is not a complete list of cautions and contraindications, so if you are unsure of anything please see your qualified healthcare professional. Plants have active phytochemicals (plant chemicals), which can interact with medications, so it is best to check with your doctor before changing your diet or supplementing with anything. Please note that in lower culinary amounts spices are generally considered safe. When they are taken in larger, more therapeutic doses there are contraindications and cautions that need to be considered. Cautions and contraindications include:

- **Anise:** Should be cautioned by pregnant women due to its emmenagogue actions.
- **Asafetida:** Should be cautioned by pregnant women due to its emmenagogue actions.
- **Chili:** Chili can burn the skin, eyes, and mucous membranes. Capsaicin cream should not be used by pregnant or breastfeeding women. Always wash hands after handling chili.
- **Cinnamon:** Never inhale cinnamon.
- **Cocoa:** Cocoa can be too stimulating (due to caffeine content) for children, so use carob powder instead, which has a similar taste, with a bit of a malty flavor.
- **Garlic:** If eaten raw, and on an empty stomach, it may cause nausea if not eaten with food. Caution to those on heart, blood pressure, and cholesterol medications, and anticoagulant medications.
- **Hibiscus:** Hibiscus should not be used during pregnancy or by those looking to conceive.
- **Licorice:** Licorice is contraindicated in high blood pressure as it can increase blood pressure. Licorice is best

used at short intervals and as professionally prescribed, if not used as a food.

- **Nutmeg:** Nutmeg should only be used in small amounts, such as a few shavings of fresh whole nutmeg or a sprinkle of nutmeg powder in cooking.
- **Peppermint:** Peppermint is contraindicated in reflux, GORD, and GERD.
- **Rose:** Do not consume or use the seeds of rose hips as they are toxic.
- **Rosemary:** Rosemary decreases iron absorption due to tannin content, so do not take with iron supplements.
- **Star anise:** Japanese star anise (*Illicium anisatum*) is a different plant to star anise (*Illicium verum*), though they look similar. Japanese star anise is toxic, so look for the correct star anise (*Illicium verum*) when purchasing.

General Information on Popular Spices

The following is a list of common spices and their uses, as well as their common name, family of origin, and the part of the spice or herb used.

Ajowan

BOTANICAL NAME: *Trachyspermum ammi, Carum ajowan*
OTHER NAMES: carom, ajwain, and ajwan
FAMILY: Apiaceae
PART USED: seed

Ajowan can be used a digestion-improving spice and as a remedy to combat an upset stomach. Ajowan has a similar taste and aroma to thyme because of its thymol essential oil content. It can be sprinkled on top of bread before baking or boiled in water as a tea. It is also sold in a special Ayurveda formula called omam water to help soothe the digestive system and reduce tummy upset.

Allspice
BOTANICAL NAME: *Pimenta dioica*
OTHER NAMES: pimento, Jamaica pepper, pimenta
FAMILY: Myrtaceae
PART USED: seed

Traditionally, allspice has been used for digestive complaints, as an aphrodisiac, as an anodyne, and for nerve pain (neuralgia). It can be used much like cloves, due to similar analgesic properties. Other potential properties of allspice include antifungal, antimicrobial, nematicidial, antidiabetic, and anticancer. Allspice berries are usually found dried as whole berries or as a powder. They can be used to flavor mulled wine, Christmas cakes, to marinate meat, and in baking. You can add allspice to flavor chai.

Aniseed
BOTANICAL NAME: *Pimpinella anisum*
OTHER NAMES: anise
FAMILY: Apiaceae, Umbelliferae
PARTS USED: fruit, seeds

Traditionally aniseed has been used as an expectorant, as a digestive tonic, to relieve heartburn, as an emmenagogue (herbs that stimulate blood flow in the pelvic area and uterus), a galactagogue (stimulates flow of mother's breast milk), and an aphrodisiac.

According to clinical nutritionist Amanda Henham, aniseed can be used "when you make a traditional chai (without the milk). You can add a few other beautiful spices, and then gently press the spices with a mortar and pestle, and add some hot water. Steep the mixture in a teapot for five minutes. And then sip away. It is also nice with fenugreek, fennel, and cinnamon."

Asafetida (pronounced "as-a-fet-i-da")

BOTANICAL NAME: *Ferula asafoetida*
OTHER NAMES: asafoetida
FAMILY: Umbelliferae
PART USED: oleo gum resin

Asafetida has been used in many traditional medicine systems including Ayurveda and Unani, and those of Afghanistan and China. Asafetida is a stimulating expectorant, antispasmodic (reduces spasms), carminative, laxative, sedative, vermifuge, diuretic, anthelmintic (herbs that expel parasitic worms), an aphrodisiac, and an emmenagogue.

It has been used in conditions such as asthma, high blood pressure, nervous conditions, bronchitis, and whooping cough. Asafetida can be found as a chunk of resin or as a powder. It is an Indian spice with an onion-like flavor. It goes well with meals that contain vegetables or mushrooms, or in curries. It can also be used on meats before frying or barbecuing. Asafetida can be used as an ingredient to help decrease flatulence when cooking beans and legumes.

Bay Leaf

BOTANICAL NAME: *Laurus nobilis*
FAMILY: Lauraceae
PART USED: leaf

Bay leaf has been found to have antioxidant properties and has been used to treat digestive issues, according to a 2006 study in the *Journal of the Iranian Chemical Society*. Bay leaf can be added to chai for a greater depth of flavor. Originally used in Mediterranean-style cooking and cuisine, the bay leaf can be used to cook broths and soups. You can cook bay leaf when cooking garlic and onions to infuse them with the flavor of bay leaf as well.

Black Pepper

BOTANICAL NAME: *Piper nigrum*
FAMILY: Piperaceae
PARTS USED: seed, fruit

Pepper's main constituents include piperine. Pepper is used for its digestive properties such as antispasmodic, carminative (herbs that prevent or treat excess gas), digestive stimulant, and possible antidiarrheal. It is also a good herb for the immune system when used as an expectorant. It is a pungent spice that is thought to be an antioxidant, anticancer, diuretic, antipyretic (fever reducer), and cholesterol lowering. It works synergistically with other herbs and spices, including turmeric, and helps increase the digestion and absorption of these herbs and spices. Black pepper is helpful for the common cold and flu, poor circulation, and poor digestion.

Black pepper can be used whole or ground fresh and used as garnish on most meals and meat. Whole peppercorns can be used as a seasoning in meals and can complement almost every savory meal. Black pepper can be used as a digestive and immune-enhancing spice ingredient in chai.

Calendula

BOTANICAL NAME: *Calendula officinalis*
FAMILY: Asteraceae
PARTS USED: flowers, petals

Calendula, also known as marigold, reduces inflammation as an anti-inflammatory flower, and is also antibacterial, lymphatic, and a great wound healer. It is suited for inflammatory skin conditions such as eczema, as well as infections and lymphatic congestion. Calendula flowers can be found fresh or dried as a tea. Fresh calendula petals can be added to salads for a vibrant pop of color. You can make calendula into a tea as infusion, into a syrup, or add it to a herbal butter. The petals can be sugared or candied and used to decorate cakes. Calendula petals can be used as a substitute to saffron when cooking rice.

Caraway

BOTANICAL NAME: *Carum carvi*
FAMILY: Apiaceae
PART USED: seed

Caraway is a carminative seed used to soothe the digestive system.

In his *Complete Herbal*, Nicholas Culpeper describes caraway as having a "moderate sharp quality, whereby it breaks wind, and provokes urine . . . it is pleasant and comfortable in the stomach, and helps digestion." Caraway can be bought as a dry seed and is delicious in German rye bread. You can make an infusion with the caraway seed or you can chew them.

Chili Pepper Varieties and Paprika

BOTANICAL NAMES: Capsicum species including *Capsicum annum, Capsicum frutescens, Capsicum chinense,* and *Capsicum pubescens*; paprika is in the same family as chili

OTHER NAMES: chile

FAMILY: Solanceae

PARTS USED: fruit, seed

Chili has a range of actions: It is a peripheral circulatory stimulant, antispasmodic, a stimulant (local and general), mucolytic, and rubefacient (topically). It can be used in cases of spasms, cramps, sore muscles, poor circulation, and for those with a "cold" constitution, meaning they have a greater tendency to feel cold.

Chili can be used fresh, as dried flakes, or a powder. The fruit and the seeds can be used in food and cooking to add extra heat. Chili goes well with savory dishes such as curries, stews, casseroles, and soups. A little bit of chili adds a good kick to sweet dishes, for example, those that feature chocolate, and in drink recipes such as the Bloody Mary cocktail. Dried chili can be infused into oil to flavor it and preserve the chili. Star anise can also be added to infused chili oil. Dried chili is often added to spice mixes and pastes. An extract of chili, capsaicin, can be found in some creams that are used topically for sore, fatigued muscles.

Paprika can be found in smoked and "sweet" varieties. Paprika goes well with red meat in stews and curries.

Cinnamon

BOTANICAL NAME: true Ceylon cinnamon (*Cinnamomum zeylanicum, Cinnamomum verum*); Chinese cassia (*Cinnamomum aromaticum Ness, Cinnamomum cassia*)

FAMILY: Lauraceae

PART USED: bark

Cinnamon is slightly sweet and bitter in taste and is a warming aromatic spice. It is astringent, mucilaginous, and antibacterial. Cinnamon is indicated in insulin resistance, diabetes mellitus, and can be used as a chest liniment. Cinnamon can be bought as a whole cinnamon stick

BOTANICAL NAME: *Syzygium aromaticum*
FAMILY: Myrtaceae
PART USED: flower buds

Clove is considered to be analgesic (pain-relieving), antibacterial, and antispasmodic. It is often used for toothache. You can buy cloves whole or as a dried powder. Cloves are an important ingredient and the predominant flavor in the South African "farmer sausage," called Boerewors.

Cocoa/Cacao

BOTANICAL NAME: *Theobroma cacao*
FAMILY: Malvaceae
PARTS USED: seed, oil

Cocoa contains antioxidants called flavonoids and polyphenols. Cocoa is also stimulating due to its caffeine and theobromine (bitter alkaloid) content. Cocoa can be cooked with a variety of sweet and savory dishes. Classically milk is used along with cocoa to make chocolate. Dark chocolate is high in cocoa content. Cocoa butter or oil is great for dry skin.

Coriander

BOTANICAL NAME: *Coriandrum sativum*
OTHER NAMES: cilantro
FAMILY: Apiaceae, Umbelliferae
PARTS USED: seed, greens

Coriander seed can be used as a carminative. You can find coriander seeds whole or as a powder. You can use the seeds in curries, spices mixes, soups, and stews. Coriander seeds can be prepared by first toasting them in a pan and then crushing or grinding them. They can add an extra flavor to Indian chai as well.

Cumin

BOTANICAL NAME: *Cuminum cyminum*
FAMILY: Umbelliferae
PART USED: seed

Cumin is antioxidant-rich and is suitable for the digestive system. Cumin is also known as *jeera* in Hindi. Cumin can be bought as a whole seed or crushed powder. The seeds and powder can be used in Indian curries and other spice mixes. It pairs well with mustard seed in curries. Ground cumin can be used to flavor dahl dishes such as red lentils (parippu), thoor dahl, etc.

Curry Leaf

BOTANICAL NAME: *Murraya koenigii*
FAMILY: Rutaceae
PART USED: leaf

According to the *Asian Journal of Pharmaceutical and Clinical Research*, curry leaves have been used as an anthelmintic (expels parasitic worms), tonic, stomachic (assists in digestions), carminative, analgesic, to reduce dysentery, to stop vomiting, and to reduce heat, inflammation, and itching. The curry leaf has been used in South Indian and Sri Lankan Tamil cooking for a long time. Curry leaf might be found as a fresh leaf at some gardening shops, although it's easy to find the dried leaf at most supermarkets.

due to its actions as an antispasmodic and digestive spice. You can buy dill seed whole, but dill leaves are often used in cooking such as in soups. It can also be used for baking bread. Dill seed, along with mustard seed, can be used to ferment or preserve pickles, and is great when used to cook fish.

Fennel

Botanical name: *Foeniculum vulgare*
Family: Apiaceae
Part used: seed

Fennel is a carminative. It also has anti-inflammatory, aromatic, antimicrobial, and diuretic properties. It is especially good for reducing flatulence. You can find fennel as a whole seed or a powder. It has a familiar "anise" flavor and is an important ingredient in curries. Fennel can be dry roasted in a sauté pan until fragrant and brown. It can then be crushed into a powder and added at the end of cooking such as in chicken, lamb, goat, or beef curry dishes. This will enhance the flavor of the curry dish. It can also be used in seafood dishes. Use ½–1 teaspoon of this mixture, mix it well through the curry, and remove the dish from the heat.

Fenugreek

BOTANICAL NAME: *Trigonella foenum-graecum*
FAMILY: Fabaceae
PART USED: seed

Fenugreek is a galactagogue (helps nursing mothers with breast milk production), it is also an expectorant, and it helps regulate blood sugar, cure constipation because of its mucilage content, and reduce digestive upset. You can find fenugreek as the whole seed. Fenugreek is often used in Indian curries. You can use fenugreek seed when you cook fish and vegetables curries. Use only ½ teaspoon, otherwise it can become bitter. It goes well with an eggplant curry. As a galactagogue, fenugreek is boiled with garlic and water and drunk in the morning during pregnancy. The green tops of fenugreek (dried), *methi*, can be used in chapati dough and in lentil dahl dishes.

Galangal

Botanical names: *Alpinia galanga, Languas galanga, Alpinia officinarum*
OTHER NAMES: *lengkuas*, which is the Malaysian word for galangal
FAMILY: Zingiberaceae
PART USED: rhizome, or root

Galangal can be used to soothe digestion as a carminative. You can buy galangal as the dried root or as a paste and you can add it to make many types of Asian-inspired soups or stocks.

Garlic

BOTANICAL NAME: *Allium sativum*
FAMILY: Amaryllidaceae
PART USED: cloves (bulb)

Garlic was used in ancient Egypt and is native to Asia. It has long been thought to be antibacterial, antiseptic, a circulatory stimulant, diaphoretic, diuretic, and antimicrobial. It can be used for high cholesterol, high blood pressure, common colds, and the flu.

BOTANICAL NAME: *Zingiber officinale*
FAMILY: Zingiberaceae
PART USED: rhizome/root

Ginger has been used in traditional Chinese medicine, Ayurveda, and Western herbal medicine. Ginger can be used as an anti-inflammatory, stimulant, diaphoretic, anodyne (reduces pain in the gastrointestinal tract and warms and stimulates the stomach), and as a rubefacient (increase blood circulation on skin). It's best for poor peripheral circulation and poor appetite, dysmenorrhoea (period pain), extreme exhaustion, flatulence and nausea, acute colds, rheumatism, and arthritic conditions. Ginger can be bought as fresh ginger rhizome or as a dried powder, which has a more intense flavor. Ginger can also be found as a syrup or crystallized. Fresh ginger can be simmered to make a decoction, or it can be infused with hot water for a simple herbal tea. Dried ginger is the key ingredient in gingerbread. It goes well with cinnamon, clove, cardamom, and nutmeg. Ginger can be made into candied ginger as a remedy to aid in reducing nausea or motion sickness. You can add ginger to many types of soups, stews, casseroles, and curries.

Green Cardamom

BOTANICAL NAME: *Elettaria cardamomum*
FAMILY: Zingiberaceae
PART USED: seed

Cardamom is a great spice to soothe digestion. Cardamom pods are usually found as whole seeds or as a powder. Naturopath Samantha Marks says, "cardamom is so versatile and can be used in sweet dishes, such as ice cream, yogurt, and cakes, and savory foods. Try it in rice pilafs and *chili con carne*. You can also use cardamom in beverages such as chai or as sugar syrup or infused alcohol. You can leave crushed pods in sugar or mix with peppercorns in a grinder to create your own Middle Eastern–inspired seasoning or add to dukah."

Cardamom can be added to tea and coffee as well. In an espresso coffeemaker or French press, brew your coffee as per your usual method, adding a cracked cardamom pod and a pinch of salt per cup before brewing. Add milk and sugar to your liking. Black cardamom, although botanically different, can also be used in certain Indian curries.

Green Tea

BOTANICAL NAME: *Camellia sinensis*
FAMILY: Theaceae
PART USED: leaves

Green tea is stimulating and calming, due to its caffeine and theanine content, respectively. It is also nootropic, and antioxidant-rich. There are many types of green tea including fermented and unfermented varieties, which all have their own unique flavors. Specific forms of green tea, such as matcha, in the form of a powder, can be used to flavor and color lattes, cakes, and ice cream. It can also be used as a broth to cook rice.

Hibiscus and Roselle
Botanical names: Hibiscus, *Hibiscus rosa-sinensis*; Roselle, *Hibiscus sabdariffa*
FAMILY: Malvaceae
PART USED: dried calyx

Horseradish
BOTANICAL NAME: *Armoracia rusticana*
FAMILY: Brassicaceae
PART USED: root

Horseradish is a mucolytic, a circulatory stimulant, and can be used in sinusitis and mucus congestion. Horseradish is classically added to cream to make horseradish cream, which can be served alongside meat. Often it is substituted for a cheaper version for what is known as wasabi paste. It can be eaten in salads or as a condiment.

Juniper Berries

BOTANICAL NAME: *Juniperus communis*
FAMILY: Cupressaceae
PART USED: berries

Juniper berries are antiseptic, stimulant, carminative, and a general diuretic. Juniper berries are usually found whole and dried. It is an essential ingredient in gin alcohol. Gin recipes vary after the main ingredient juniper berry. Botanical herbs and spices such as angelica root and coriander seed are used in gin, as well as lemon peel. Juniper berries are also delicious studded into pieces of meat and then pan-cooked.

Licorice

BOTANICAL NAME: *Glycyrrhiza glabra*
FAMILY: Fabaceae
PART USED: root

Licorice has been found as an anti-inflammatory, mucilaginous, antiviral, and anti-androgenic. It can be used for sore, dry throats, colds and flus, nervous exhaustion, stress, fatigue, androgen-related acne, to soothe the stomach and gastrointestinal lining, and to aid *H. pylori* eradication. Herbalists may prescribe a deglycyrrhizinated form of licorice (DGL). Licorice root can be bought as milled root that can be made into a decoction. It is generally found in the form of the dried root or as a tea mix, on its own, or mixed with other herbs or spices. Licorice goes well with other warm spices such as cinnamon, ginger, and cloves. It also goes well with chocolate.

Mustard

BOTANICAL NAMES: yellow mustard (*Brassica alba*), brown mustard (*Brassica juncea*), and black mustard (*Brassica nigra*)
FAMILY: Brassicaceae
PART USED: seed

Mustard has been known to act as a counter-stimulant on the skin and a warming circulating stimulant in the body. Mustard can be used as a poultice and as part of a mustard footbath. There are various kinds of mustard seeds in the Brassicaceae family such as yellow, black, and brown seeds. Small mustard seeds can be used in a variety of Indian dishes. Mustard seeds are used to make various kinds of mustard spreads and sauces.

Myrrh

BOTANICAL NAME: *Commiphora myrrha*
FAMILY: Burseraceae
PART USED: resin

Myrrh is anti-inflammatory, wound healing, astringent, and antiseptic. It is helpful for treating sore, dry throats, sore mouths, and ulcers, and is great for improving skin conditions. It can also be used as a throat gargle. Myrrh can be used on the skin to reduce inflammation and encourage skin healing. Myrrh has traditionally been used as a perfume and as incense.

Nigella seed

BOTANICAL NAME: *Nigella sativa*
OTHER NAMES: black seed, black cumin, kalonji
FAMILY: Ranunculaceae
PART USED: seeds

Nigella seed is an immune modulator, anti-inflammatory, a digestive aid, and has antiseptic properties. It is also helpful for weight loss, low immune system function, and poor digestion.

It is found as the whole black seed, which can be used in salads much like other nuts. The seed oil can also be used in salad dressings. Nigella seed can be used in curries, can be sprinkled on top of bread, and can be used when making naan. It can be tempered in oil before adding meat to cook.

Nutmeg and Mace

BOTANICAL NAME: *Myristica fragrans*

FAMILY: Myristicaceae

PART USED: seed (nutmeg) and the aril
surrounding the seed (mace)

While nutmeg is generally only used as food flavoring these days, herbalist Nicholas Culpeper believed that nutmeg could "strengthen the brain, stomach, and liver, ease the pain of the spleen, stop looseness, ease pains of the head and pains in the joints, strengthen the body, take away weakness coming of cold, and cause a sweet breath." Nutmeg has been thought to be antiemetic, carminative, spasmolytic, orexigenic (appetite stimulant), a gastric secretion stimulant, an inhibitor of prostaglandin, and an aphrodisiac. Mace is the outer covering of nutmeg, which is extracted for its specific uses and used in cooking.

Nutmeg is best used in cooking in only small amounts. Nutmeg can be bought as a whole nutmeg, which retains its flavor more than a powder does. It can be grated from a whole nutmeg as a garnish, on egg-based desserts, and into eggnog. Nutmeg is delicious when used in marinades for meat, before being cooked. It is a key flavor used to make "jerk" chicken and apple strudel. You can temper whole mace with spices such as cinnamon quill, star anise, cloves, or cardamom pods before adding to dishes such as those of Malaysian origin.

Onion

BOTANICAL NAME: *Allium cepa*
FAMILY: Amaryllidaceae
PART USED: bulb

Onion has been known to be a mucolytic, anti-inflammatory, and antibacterial, and has been used for the common cold, influenza, for sore throats, and for general immune system health. Onions can be bought fresh as whole bulbs, pickled, and also as dried granules. They are one of the most versatile foods and flavorings. Dried onions can be mixed into ground beef before forming burgers, and pickled onion can be added to Vietnamese banh mi. Onions combine well with garlic, and can be pickled in vinegar or fermented in a brine for storage.

Peppermint

BOTANICAL NAME: *Mentha piperita*
FAMILY: Lamiaceae (mint)
PART USED: leaves

Peppermint is antibacterial, antispasmodic, carminative, stomachic, a stimulant, a local anesthetic (e.g., to relieve pain from rheumatism and inflammation), and it is cooling because of menthol. Peppermint is good for the common cold, influenza, managing fevers, reducing inflammation in the throat, relieving toothaches, and as a cooling mouthwash. In the digestive system, peppermint is used for conditions such as colic, nausea and vomiting, spasms in the gastrointestinal tract, indigestion, to promote digestion, and in irritable bowel syndrome. You can find peppermint leaves fresh or dried. Peppermint can be added to an iced drink to cool you down, in a cold or warm infusion, and the fresh leaves can be added to salads, soups, and as a garnish on many meals.

Rose

BOTANICAL NAMES: *Rosa damascena* (Damask rose),
Rosa multiflora, Rosa rugosa, Rosa canina
FAMILY: Rosaceae
PART USED: rose petals, rose hips

Rose has been used in many traditional medicine systems including Western herbal medicine, traditional Chinese medicine, and Iranian systems of medicine. Roses that are very fragrant are generally beneficial. Rose is calming, a mild nervine, astringent and antibacterial, bactericidal, antidepressant, a heart tonic, a stomachic, and a depurative. Rose can be used during emotional upset and to calm the nervous system.

You can find roses as fresh rose petals or dried. You can use fresh or dried rose petals to make a bright and uplifting pink infusion. Rose petals are often used in food as a flavoring and a spice. The petals can be candied for cake decorations.

Roses can be kept in the garden for their gentle aroma. Rose can be extracted in the form of rose water, which is the main flavor in Turkish delights. Rose can be added into chai mixes as a flavor enhancer, and can be used in Middle Eastern cooking in a variety of dishes. Dried roses can be used in potpourri mixes and in body products. Rose can also be made into a sweet jam or jelly or bought as an essential oil to use in an oil burner. Always buy organic when buying roses for consumption or using externally to avoid pesticide exposure.

Rosemary

BOTANICAL NAME: *Rosmarinus officinalis*
FAMILY: Lamiaceae
PARTS USED: leaves, aerial parts

Rosemary is an antioxidant and it can aid liver detoxification. It is hepatoproctive (liver protecting), a nervine, a relaxing tonic, a peripheral circulatory stimulator, an astringent, and a diuretic. It is indicated in certain liver conditions, can help improve memory, reduce stress, and is a nootropic. Rosemary can be bought fresh and dried. It classically goes well with roasted meats and roasted root vegetables such as potatoes. It can be made into an herbal salt by blending salt with rosemary. Dried rosemary can be infused into oils for cooking or to use as salad dressings.

Saffron

BOTANICAL NAME: *Crocus sativus*
FAMILY: Iridaceae
PARTS USED: petals, green leaves, and stigmas

Saffron is potentially antiedematogenic and potentially antinociceptive (stops pain). It is thought to have anti-inflammatory properties and is used to treat depression. Some modern herbalists and naturopaths may prescribe and dispense extract of saffron if they feel it is necessary, depending on particular health circumstances and conditions. Saffron can be found as whole styles or stigmas. It is used to flavor and color rice in both sweet and savory dishes. Usually the stigmas are soaked in water and this water is added along with the stigmas to a dish to be cooked. Saffron may be quite expensive for everyday use; however, you only need to use a small amount when cooking.

Sage

BOTANICAL NAME: *Salvia officinalis*
FAMILY: Lamiaceae
PART USED: leaves

Sage is an antihyperhidrotic, antibacterial, astringent, stimulant, and carminative. It can be used for sore, dry throats (it is good also with myrrh), inflammation in the mouth and throat, menopausal hot flushes, to reduce excess sweating and perspiration, inflammation of the skin, flatulence, poor digestion, and mild dyspepsia. You can use sage to make herbal infusions, add it to soups or stews, make a mouth gargle for sore throats, or make homemade deodorant or mouth-wash along with peppermint.

Star Anise

BOTANICAL NAME: *Illicium verum*
FAMILY: Schisandraceae
PART USED: fruit

Star anise has antimicrobial properties and has traditionally been used as a carminative. You can find star anise as whole dried fruits or as a powder. You can add it to broths, soups, and stews, and it can be infused into oil. It goes well with chili and chocolate, and is used in some Asian cooking with pork and in Chinese five-spice powder.

Sumac

BOTANICAL NAME: *Rhus coriaria*
FAMILY: Anacardiaceae
PART USED: berry

Researcher Arham Shabbir (2012) explains that sumac has been used in many traditional medicine systems including in

Persia, the Mediterranean and Middle East, Turkey, Palestine, Golan Heights, Israel, and Jordan. Shabbir also notes that sumac has been shown to have antibacterial, hepatoprotective, antifungal, antioxidant, anti-inflammatory, DNA protective, anti-ischemic, and vasorelaxant activities, among other actions. Sumac has a sour taste and goes well with fish and other seafood, lamb and yogurt, and Middle Eastern dishes. You can add it to raw salads or to cooked greens. Sumac is an ingredient in Middle Eastern za'atar. You can use sumac in Lebanese-style salads.

Szechuan Pepper

BOTANICAL NAME: *Zanthoxylum simulans*
FAMILY: Rutaceae
PART USED: seed

Szechuan pepper stimulates saliva and can numb the mouth. It can be found as the whole berry and combines well with beef and Asian-style noodles. You can heat Szechuan pepper in oil until blackened and then add it to a variety of meat, noodle, and vegetable dishes. It is delicious and has a zingy flavor. You can also add Szechuan pepper to a pepper grinder along with salt and other spices and add this to your meals instead of black pepper.

Thyme

BOTANICAL NAME: *Thymus vulgaris*
FAMILY: Lamiaceae
PART USED: leaves

Thyme has antibacterial properties. It is indicated for use in colds, the flu, sore throats, and coughs. It can be cooked with mushrooms, butter, and garlic, and it is traditionally used in bouquet garni along with other herbs. It goes well on roasted meats, vegetables, and in salads.

Turmeric

BOTANICAL NAME: *Curcuma longa*
FAMILY: Zingiberaceae
PART USED: root

Turmeric is anti-inflammatory, antioxidant, and antibacterial, and it is thought to have beneficial effects in Alzheimer's. It is also a liver tonic. Turmeric can be found in grocery stores, health food shops, and farmers' markets in fresh rhizome form as well as the dried powder. Turmeric is an essential ingredient in Indian curries. Fresh turmeric can be prepared in many ways including grating it, juicing it, and sautéing grated pieces in a curry base. You can add a small amount of turmeric, about ¼–½ teaspoon, to smoothies for a nutritional boost. It can also be mixed into yogurt and added to lentils to make dahl. If you'd like, you can use it as a substitute for saffron to color rice. It can be used in some drinks such as Golden Milk (see Chapter 16) and even in chai. Black pepper can help increase the absorption of turmeric.

Vanilla

BOTANICAL NAME: *Vanilla planifolia*
FAMILY: Orchidaceae
PART USED: beans, pod, and seeds

Vanilla is thought to be an uplifting spice, often thought to be an aphrodisiac. Vanilla can be bought as an extract, bean, paste, or essence. The essence, however, is an artificial form that does not contain any real extract of vanilla. It is mostly used in sweet dishes, desserts, and drinks. After a vanilla bean has been scraped, the leftover bean pod can be put into a jar of sugar to infuse the granules with vanilla aroma and taste. Vanilla can also be made into a homemade vanilla extract. You can add vanilla to a tea along with rose petals. Vanilla can also be added to nourishing, sweet custard.

Wild Celery Seed

BOTANICAL NAME: *Apium graveolens*
FAMILY: Umbelliferae
PARTS USED: as a spice, seed; in cooking, seed and stem

Many parts of celery can be used including the stalk and the seed. Celery seed can be used as a diuretic, anti-inflammatory, and pain-reliever (as a secondary action).

Celery seed can be found whole, as a powder, and as celery salt. It can be used in spice mixes and in meat rubs.

CHAPTER 12

Breakfast

Cinnamon and Banana Smoothie

This is an easy and tasty way to start your day. The cinnamon is delicious in this recipe and it helps support healthy blood sugar levels. The banana also makes this recipe quite creamy and is a good source of soluble fiber.

INGREDIENTS | SERVES 2

1 cup full-fat or alternative milk
½ cup live Greek yogurt (or dairy-free yogurt)
1 banana, frozen and chopped
1 teaspoon *true* cinnamon root powder
1 teaspoon honey (optional)

1. Add milk, yogurt, banana, cinnamon, and honey to blender and close lid.
2. Blend on high until it becomes a smooth, creamy consistency.
3. Pour into glasses and serve.

Special Equipment

You will need a strong blender. Alternatively you can use a stick blender and a bowl to blend this smoothie together.

Poha (Rice Breakfast Dish)

Poha is flat, rolled rice. This Poha is a spiced mix of rice along with spices and fresh herbs. It is a delicious and popular breakfast dish. Rai seed are small black seeds from the mustard family that can be bought from an Indian grocery store.

INGREDIENTS | SERVES 2

2 cups poha (flat, rolled rice)
2 tablespoons olive oil
½ teaspoon cumin seed
½ teaspoon rai seed
1 medium onion, peeled and chopped
¼ teaspoon salt
½ teaspoon ground turmeric

1. Place poha in a bowl of water. Wet, and then strain. You don't want to wet it too much otherwise it can become soggy.
2. Wait 5–10 minutes and then loosen the rice to separate it a bit.
3. In a large sauté pan over medium-high heat, heat the oil and add cumin and rai seed.
4. Add the onion to the pan and cook until it is crunchy, about 4–6 minutes.
5. Add salt and turmeric. Then add the poha and cook for about 5 minutes more.

Additions

If you'd like, you can add tomatoes to this recipe for a nice acidic undertone. You can also add fresh green chili or some peanuts to the poha. Serve this with chopped raw red onion, peanuts, and fresh coriander.

Cardamom Lassi

This drink recipe can be had with breakfast, as a snack, or even alongside a spicy meal. Thanks to the yogurt and cardamom, this drink is good for those with digestive issues. You can use coconut yogurt and an alternative milk, such as coconut or almond milk, for a dairy-free version, if desired.

INGREDIENTS | SERVES 2

3 green cardamom pods
1 cup natural yogurt (or dairy-free yogurt)
¼ cup milk (or dairy-free milk)
2 ice cubes
1 teaspoon honey

1. Crush the cardamom pods to release the seeds. Discard the cardamom skins.

2. Add the seeds to a blender along with the yogurt, milk, ice, and honey.

3. Blend on high until very smooth. Serve immediately and enjoy.

Spiced Stewed Fruit

This is a nice recipe that you can serve over granola, muesli, or porridge. It can also be served as a dessert with custard or ice cream.

INGREDIENTS | SERVES 4

2 medium pears, or other seasonal stone fruit, cored and sliced
2 tablespoons (or to taste) honey
¼ teaspoon "Mixed Spice" powder
¼ teaspoon nutmeg shavings
3 cloves
⅛ teaspoon salt
¼ cup dried cranberries or sultanas

1. Add pears to a medium saucepan.

2. In a medium bowl, mix together honey, mixed spices, nutmeg, cloves, and salt. Pour this mixture into the saucepan and stir evenly. Add cranberries.

3. Turn the stove to medium-high and start to simmer the mixture. Stir and cook the mixture for about 10–15 minutes or until the pears become very soft.

Mixed Spice

You can make your own mixed spice powder with spices such as cinnamon, cloves, nutmeg, and ginger.

Toasted and Spiced Granola

This is a delicious, crunchy granola. It features vanilla and cinnamon for a bit of sweetness. It can be eaten for breakfast or it can be used as a topping on ice cream or yogurt for dessert.

INGREDIENTS | SERVES 4–6

1 cup raw honey
1 teaspoon vanilla extract
1 teaspoon ground cinnamon
2 cups rolled oats
½ cup quinoa flakes (or use rolled oats instead)
½ cup unsalted cashews
½ cup walnuts, broken in half
½ cup almonds
½ cup pepitas

1. Preheat the oven to 350°F.

2. In a small saucepan over medium heat, melt the honey gently and stir in vanilla extract.

3. Add cinnamon, oats, quinoa, nuts, and seeds and mix to coat everything evenly.

4. Spread out this mixture in a baking tray and cook about 40–45 minutes until the granola becomes dry and light brown. It is a good idea to give the granola a mix so it browns and cooks evenly. Once it is cooked, leave to cool and then store in airtight jars in the cupboard.

CHAPTER 13

Appetizers and Vegetable Side Dishes

Thyme Garlic and Pepper Mushrooms

This vegetarian recipe is delicious with breakfast, lunch, or dinner. It is also nice added to a quiche mixture and then baked.

INGREDIENTS | SERVES 1–2

1 tablespoon butter
2 cloves garlic, peeled and crushed
8 ounces button mushrooms, sliced
1 teaspoon olive oil
1 tablespoon fresh or dried thyme
¼ teaspoon salt
¼ teaspoon freshly cracked black pepper

1. To a medium sauté pan over medium heat, add butter and garlic. Heat until the garlic browns slightly, 5–8 minutes.

2. Add mushrooms, oil, thyme, and salt to the pan. Stir and heat mushrooms until they are soft and have turned a golden brown, 6–8 minutes. Serve with freshly cracked pepper.

Gobi Aloo Subji

This is a spiced, savory Indian cauliflower dish. Gobi means "cauliflower" and aloo means "potato."

INGREDIENTS | SERVES 4–6

2 teaspoons ghee or butter

1 teaspoon cumin seed

1 teaspoon ria seed

1 medium onion, peeled and chopped

½ quantity Tomato Gravy (see Chapter 14)

1 medium head cauliflower, chopped and leaves removed

2 medium potatoes, cubed

1 teaspoon turmeric powder

1 teaspoon salt, or to taste

3 cups water

1. Heat butter in a medium sauté pan over medium heat. Add cumin and ria seeds to the butter. Leave them to cook 3–5 minutes or until they start to pop.

2. Add onion and Tomato Gravy. Add cauliflower and potatoes. Stir to coat.

3. Add turmeric, salt, and 3 cups water.

4. Put a lid on the pot and leave to cook until the cauliflower is very soft, which may take about 30 minutes.

Sumac and Walnut Salad

This recipe is a nice, easy, and a delicious way to get more green leafy vegetables in your diet.

INGREDIENTS | SERVES 2–4

1 teaspoon sumac
1 tablespoon olive oil
⅛ teaspoon salt
2 cups baby spinach leaves or rocket leaves
¼ cup chopped walnuts

1. In a small bowl, mix together sumac, olive oil, and salt.
2. To a large bowl, add the spinach or rocket leaves. Pour the sumac dressing over the leaves. Top the salad with walnuts.

Spinach with Garlic and Chili

This is a delicious and simple recipe for anyone who likes a bit of heat and flavor with green leafy vegetables, or for those who need a few new ways to cook leafy greens. Serve as a side or on top of pasta.

INGREDIENTS | SERVES 2–4

1 tablespoon butter
2 cloves garlic, peeled and crushed
¼ teaspoon chili powder
5 cups baby spinach
¼ teaspoon salt

1. In a large pot over medium heat, melt butter and add garlic. Stir 4–6 minutes, making sure the butter doesn't burn, until the garlic has browned slightly.

2. Add chili powder and baby spinach. Add salt.

3. Stir the spinach into the butter mixture and cook, while stirring, for 3–4 minutes until the spinach softens and wilts.

CHAPTER 14

Lunch and Dinner

Tempered Rice

Tempered rice is a delicious way to flavor plain rice and make a curry even more interesting.

INGREDIENTS | MAKES 1 CUP

1 cup basmati rice
1½ cups water
1 tablespoon olive oil
6 fresh curry leaves
1 teaspoon cumin seeds
2 tablespoons urad dahl

1. Add rice and water to a medium saucepan. Bring to a boil over medium-high heat. Place a tight-fitting lid on the pot and then turn down the heat to very low. Cook until the water is absorbed, about 15–20 minutes.

2. Remove pot from heat and allow to sit for 10 minutes.

3. In a medium sauté pan, add olive oil over medium-high heat. Add the curry leaves and fry for 30 seconds. Be careful the oil doesn't splatter. Add the cumin and urad dahl to the curry leaf-oil mixture and fry 3–5 minutes until the urad dahl becomes golden. Stir the mixture into the rice.

Tomato Gravy

This recipe will be needed as a base for the Mung Bean Dahl. This Tomato Gravy recipe can be used to cook other lentils and beans as well.

INGREDIENTS | MAKES 2–4 CUPS

4 medium tomatoes

2 teaspoons salt

2 cloves garlic, peeled

3 teaspoons turmeric powder

Combine tomatoes, salt, garlic, and turmeric powder and blend until smooth.

Rasam (Spicy Soup)

This is a simple yet flavorful spice-based soup. This is based on a South Indian/Sri Lankan recipe. Many thanks go to Jaya for this recipe. Srijaya (Jaya) is a home cook who was born in Malaysia and is of Sri Lankan background. She has also taught cooking classes in Japan.

INGREDIENTS | YIELDS 3 CUPS

5 tablespoons coriander seed

1 tablespoon black peppercorns

2 tablespoons cumin seed

3 cups water

3 tablespoons tamarind purée or paste

5 cloves garlic, skins on and roughly pounded

¼ teaspoon salt

3 tablespoons vegetable oil

½ teaspoon black mustard seed

1 medium red onion, peeled and thinly sliced

2–3 dried chilies, torn into pieces

2 stalks curry leaves

1. In a coffee grinder or with a mortar and pestle, grind coriander, peppercorns, and cumin together until you have a powder.

2. In a medium stockpot, add water, tamarind purée, and garlic, and bring to a boil. Add the powdered spices to the pot, mix well, and bring back to a boil. Add salt and remove from heat.

3. In a medium frying pan over medium heat, heat the oil and add mustard seed. Once the mustard seed has popped, add the sliced onion and stir-fry until the onion is caramelized, about 7–9 minutes.

4. Add dried chilies and curry leaves. Fry until the curry leaves are fragrant, about 3–5 minutes. Pour this mixture into the stockpot and stir.

Variations

If you'd like, you can add lentils to this soup. Put 3–4 tablespoon of red lentils with water, tamarind purée, and garlic and bring to a boil in stockpot. Reduce the heat and simmer until the lentils are cooked, about 15–20 minutes, or until lentils are very soft. Also, adding 2–3 freshly diced tomatoes makes this soup more robust and tangy. You can also add chopped fresh cilantro as garnish, if preferred.

Chole

For this recipe, if you are short on time, you can also use canned (precooked) and well-drained chickpeas instead of dried chickpeas.

INGREDIENTS | SERVES 4 AS A SIDE DISH

1 cup dried chickpeas
3 cups water
1 medium onion, peeled and finely chopped
1 tablespoon olive oil
1 tablespoon cumin powder
1 tablespoon turmeric powder
1 tablespoon finely chopped fresh garlic
1 tablespoon finely chopped ginger
1–2 cups chicken or vegetable stock
½ cup tomato paste
¼ teaspoon salt
3 medium white potatoes, peeled and cubed

1. Add chickpeas to a large stockpot filled with enough water to cover them. Bring to a boil and then simmer chickpeas over medium-high heat until they are very soft, about 3–4 hours; however, you can speed this up by using a pressure cooker or by using canned (and drained) chickpeas. Canned chickpeas will only take about 30 minutes. Drain and put aside.

2. In a large sauté pan over medium heat, fry onion in oil until translucent, about 3–5 minutes. Add cumin and turmeric powder, and fry for 1 minute. Add garlic and ginger. Add stock and tomato paste. Mix.

3. Add chickpeas and stir. Add salt.

4. Add potatoes and cook 5–8 minutes or until tender. Add more stock as required.

Basic Indian-Style Curry with Lamb

This is a good basic recipe for curries. Lamb has been used in this curry. If you don't want to use meat, you can use tofu, beans, or vegetables instead.

INGREDIENTS | SERVES 2–4

1 tablespoon olive oil
1 medium onion, peeled and chopped
1 teaspoon cumin seed
1 tablespoon garam masala
1 teaspoon turmeric powder
¼ teaspoon chili powder (optional)
1 teaspoon salt
1 teaspoon granulated sugar
1 teaspoon garlic-ginger paste (homemade or store-bought)
1 cup chicken stock, plus extra as needed
14 ounces canned diced tomatoes
2 pounds lamb (or root vegetables or tofu)

1. Add oil and onion to a large sauté pan. Fry onion over medium heat for 3–5 minutes, and then add cumin seed.

2. Add garam masala, turmeric, and chili powder (if using), and fry 1 minute.

3. Add salt, sugar, garlic-ginger paste, chicken stock, and tomatoes.

4. Cook tomato mixture until it thickens into a paste-like consistency, up to 20 minutes. Make sure to stir so the mixture doesn't burn.

5. Let it simmer 1–2 hours on very low heat.

6. Now add meat (or vegetables) and cook on low until the meat (or vegetables) is tender and cooked through (make sure lamb reaches 145°F.

7. You may need to add additional stock as the sauce condenses down.

Vegetable Variation

If you are making a vegetable-only curry, the sauce needs to be cooked a little longer and be reasonably thick before adding the vegetables compared to a meat-based curry. This is because vegetables cook more quickly than meat.

Jaya's Rendang Curry

Thank you to Jaya for this delicious Malaysian Rendang Curry recipe. You can make the paste, or the whole curry, ahead, to cook later or serve when you're ready, respectively.

INGREDIENTS | SERVES 8

Spice Paste

5 shallots or 2 large onions, peeled and chopped

1" piece galangal, chopped

3 stalks lemongrass (the white part only), cut into small pieces

5 cloves garlic, peeled and crushed

1" piece ginger, chopped

10–12 dried, whole red hot peppers (chilies) (soaked in warm water, seeded, and strained before using) or 2 tablespoons red chili powder

Toasted Coconut

1 cup dried coconut

Curry

1 tablespoon olive oil or ghee

1 stick cinnamon

3 cloves

3 star anise

3 cardamom pods, pounded slightly

2 pounds diced beef or lamb with bones

1 or 2 stalks lemongrass, cut into 4" pieces and pounded slightly

1 (13.5-ounce) can coconut milk

2 teaspoons tamarind paste

1 cup water

6 kaffir lime leaves

1 tablespoon brown sugar or palm sugar

¼ teaspoon salt

1. Add the spice paste ingredients to a food processor and process until a fine paste is produced. Put this aside and clean and dry the food processor.

2. In a dry wok or small sauté pan over low heat, slowly toast the dried coconut until very dark, deep brown and fragrant (but not black or burnt), which will take about 10–12 minutes. It will need to be stirred frequently. Allow to cool.

3. Once the coconut is cooled, add to food processor, coffee grinder, or mortar and pestle, and grind until it becomes a rough consistency. Put aside.

4. In a wok or large stockpot, heat the oil over medium-high heat and sauté cinnamon, cloves, star anise, and cardamom until aromatic, about 5–8 minutes.

5. Add spice paste. Stir until fragrant and the oil rises to the surface, about 5 minutes, and the mixture takes on a sauce-like consistency. Keep stirring the mixture so it doesn't burn. You may want to add a bit more water if it gets too dry.

6. Add diced meat and lemongrass to paste mixture. Stir until well coated with paste, continuously stirring 1–2 minutes. Add coconut milk, tamarind paste, and water.

7. Simmer on medium heat, stirring frequently, until meat is almost cooked, about 8 minutes. Add kaffir lime leaves, coconut, and sugar, and stir until well coated with sauce.

8. Lower heat to low. Cover with a lid and let simmer for 1–1½ hours, or until the meat is tender and the gravy has thickened up. Occasionally open and stir the mixture so that the mixture does not burn at the bottom.

9. Once the meat is tender, add salt. If it is not sweet enough, add extra sugar. Discard the lemongrass stalks and serve.

Curry Variations

Using dried chilies produces a hotter curry, while using chili powder creates a slightly less hot curry, but one with a brighter, redder color. If you'd like, after the spice paste and toasted coconut are made, this curry can be cooked in a slow cooker. Instead of warm rice or glutinous rice, this can be served with "ghee rice," which is rice that has been sautéed with spices and ghee. Biryani rice is also nice with this dish.

Immune-Boosting Asian Chicken Soup

Chicken soup is used in many cultures as an immune-boosting tonic for vitality and wellness. This broth takes inspiration from traditional Chinese medicine with the use of goji berries, astragalus root, ginger, and garlic. This soup is ideal to use preventively, for colds and flus.

INGREDIENTS | YIELDS 10–12 CUPS

1 (2-pound) raw chicken carcass

12 cups water

1 tablespoon apple cider vinegar

1 piece dried astragalus root (known as huang qi), soaked in 1 cup water

1 medium brown onion, peeled and chopped

1 tablespoon sliced ginger

2 cloves garlic, peeled and chopped (reserve peels)

1 cup goji berries (also known as wolf-berries), divided

¼ teaspoon salt

1. Add chicken to a large stockpot and cover with 12 cups water, making sure the water level is above the chicken. Add a bit more water if needed. Bring to a boil over medium-high heat. Lower heat to medium-low, and bring to a simmer.

2. Add vinegar, astragalus, onion (along with the peels), ginger, and garlic.

3. Simmer 1–3 hours, or longer if possible, for up to 12 hours, as this helps extract the nutrients from all the ingredients into the broth.

4. Strain the mixture to remove the chicken carcass, astragalus, onion, onion peels, ginger, and garlic (you can keep the onion, ginger, and garlic in the soup if you like).

5. Add about 1–2 teaspoons goji berries to each bowl of soup before serving. Season each bowl with salt.

Salty Soup

It is best to avoid putting salt in the soup until the very end of this recipe, as this mixture can condense and the soup can be become too salty.

Szechuan Pepper Chicken and Noodle Soup

You can use this recipe (minus the rice noodles) in place of regular stock or broth in any recipe for a natural immune boost!

INGREDIENTS | SERVES 2

2 tablespoons olive oil, divided
1 tablespoon dried Szechuan pepper berries
2 (4-ounce) chicken breasts, sliced into long strips
1 onion, peeled and thinly sliced
3 cloves garlic, 2 peeled and crushed, 1 chopped into small pieces, divided
1 knob of ginger, sliced
1 small red chili, sliced and seeds removed
2 cups chicken stock or broth
1 large bunch Asian greens, chopped
2 ounces dried rice noodles

1. Heat a large stockpot over medium heat and add 1 tablespoon oil.

2. Add Szechuan pepper and heat while stirring until fragrant and the berries have blackened, about 5 minutes. You can choose to keep the Szechuan peppers in for a bit of crunch or you can strain them out to keep just the oil.

3. Add chicken and cook until all edges have browned slightly, 6–8 minutes.

4. Turn heat to medium-low; add onion, garlic, and ginger, and cook until the onion is translucent, about 5 minutes.

5. Add chili and stock or broth. Add Asian greens and put a lid on the pot. Allow to simmer over medium heat for about 15–20 minutes.

6. In a separate medium stockpot, boil rice noodles until tender. Once well cooked, strain and divide the noodles into 2 bowls.

7. Divide the chicken soup into the bowls and enjoy.

Mung Bean Dahl

There are two parts for this recipe: the first is the Tomato Gravy (see recipe in this chapter) and the second part is the cooking of the dahl. First make the Tomato Gravy, which becomes the base of the dahl. Then you will use the Tomato Gravy to cook the Mung Bean Dahl.

INGREDIENTS | SERVES 4–6, AS A SIDE DISH

1 cup dried mung beans

4 cups water, divided

1 tablespoon butter

1 tablespoon oil

1 teaspoon cumin seed

1 teaspoon ria seed (small black mustard seed)

2 cups Tomato Gravy (see recipe in this chapter)

1. Add mung beans, 2 cups water, and butter to a 4–6-quart pressure cooker. Cook at medium heat until the mung beans have become very soft, about 10–15 minutes.

2. In a medium sauté pan, heat oil over medium heat and add cumin and ria seeds. Cook for 4–6 minutes, or until the seeds start to pop. Make sure they don't burn.

3. Add Tomato Gravy. Add mung bean mixture and 2 cups water. Cook about 5 minutes longer. Serve hot.

Charakku Curry Powder

The spices in this recipe can help aid in digestion and infection recovery. Thank you to Srijaya Sriharan for sharing this recipe.

INGREDIENTS | MAKES ABOUT 1 CUP

18 tablespoons (9 ounces) coriander seed

3 teaspoons black peppercorns

2 teaspoons fenugreek seed

2 teaspoons cumin seed

8 teaspoons fennel seed

2 teaspoons black mustard seed

5–7 curry leaves, finely sliced

½" piece turmeric root

2 teaspoons uncooked parboiled rice

1. Wash coriander, peppercorns, fenugreek, cumin, and fennel seeds separately and sun-dry well. Dry roast spices (but not the mustard seeds) by adding spices to a dry pan over medium-high heat and heating 5–8 minutes until aromatic. Remove from pan and set aside.

2. In the same pan, dry roast curry leaves with coriander and turmeric root over medium-high heat about 5–8 minutes until aromatic.

3. Mix all the ingredients together, including the uncooked parboiled rice. In a coffee grinder, grind the mixed spices, leaves, turmeric root, and rice until it forms a powder. Store in an airtight container.

Chicken Charakku Curry

It's best to serve this chicken curry with rice to subdue the spices.

INGREDIENTS | SERVES 4

½ pound boneless and skinless chicken thighs, cut into bite-sized pieces
1 large onion, peeled and diced
1 dried whole red chili
¼ teaspoon fenugreek seed
6 whole cloves garlic, peeled
⅛ teaspoon turmeric powder
¼ teaspoon salt
2 cups water, divided
3–4 tablespoons Charakku Curry Powder (see recipe in this chapter)
½ teaspoon tamarind paste
6–8 curry leaves
1 tablespoon thick coconut cream

1. In a large stockpot, add chicken pieces, onion, chili, fenugreek, garlic, turmeric, salt, and 1½ cups water. Bring to a boil over medium-high heat.

2. In a small bowl, mix curry powder, tamarind, and ½ cup water into a paste.

3. Add paste mixture, curry leaves, and coconut cream to the stockpot and return to a boil. Simmer 2 minutes and remove from heat. Serve hot.

Vegetarian Charakku Curry

This is a vegetarian version of the Chicken Charakku Curry. Serve with rice.

INGREDIENTS | SERVES 4

½ pound vegetables (baby eggplants, ash plantain, or potatoes), cut into bite-sized pieces

1 large onion, peeled and diced

1 dried red (chili) pepper

6 cloves garlic, peeled and crushed

⅛ teaspoon turmeric powder

¼ teaspoon fenugreek seed

¼ teaspoon salt

2 cups water, divided

2–3 tablespoon Charakku Curry Powder (see recipe in this chapter)

½ teaspoon tamarind purée or paste

6–8 curry leaves

1 tablespoon thick coconut cream

1. In a large stockpot over medium-high heat, add vegetables, onion, chili, garlic, turmeric, fenugreek, salt, and 1½ cups water. Cover and cook until vegetables are tender, about 30–40 minutes.

2. In a small bowl, mix curry powder, tamarind, and ½ cup water into a paste.

3. Add paste mixture, curry leaves, and coconut cream to the stockpot and bring to a boil. Remove from heat and serve hot.

CHAPTER 15

Condiments, Rubs, and Marinades

Chili Oil

This is a condiment for those of you who like a little bit of bite in your meals. A meal without Chili Oil is not the same. Chili Oil can also be added during cooking.

INGREDIENTS | MAKES 1 CUP

¾ cup dried, crushed red pepper (chili) flakes
1 cup olive oil

1. Add chili flakes to a sterile Mason jar. Add olive oil slowly, allowing the chili flakes to absorb the oil before adding more. Add all the oil to the jar.

2. Leave to infuse for a few days on the counter. Keep stored in a cupboard away from sunlight.

Ginger and Garlic Paste

Ginger and Garlic Paste is a staple in many Indian and Asian dishes. You can make as much or as little of this paste as you'd like, but just be sure to use the ratio of 1 part ginger to 2 parts garlic.

INGREDIENTS | MAKES 1½ CUPS

½ cup roughly chopped fresh ginger

1 cup peeled and chopped garlic cloves

1. Add ginger and garlic to a small blender or food processor. Blend until a smooth paste forms.

2. Store in a lidded glass jar in the refrigerator.

Homemade Vanilla Extract

You can make vanilla extract very easily at home. It also tastes much more flavorful than store-bought vanilla extract and it can be made sugar- and/or alcohol-free if you wish—just replace the alcohol with glycerin. Glycerin is naturally sweet but does not contain any sugar. Use this in baked goods, hot drinks, cold drinks, and ice cream.

INGREDIENTS | MAKES 1¼ CUPS

¾ cup glycerin

¼ cup water

¼ cup vodka

6–8 vanilla beans, sliced in half lengthwise and cut into small pieces

1. Add glycerin, water, and vodka to a wide-mouth glass jar and mix together with a spoon.

2. Add the cut vanilla beans to the jar.

3. Put the lid on the jar and give the vanilla extract a good shake. Label the jar with "vanilla extract" and the date you made it.

4. Leave the jar in a dark cupboard about 4–6 weeks or until the extract tastes strongly of vanilla. Shake it every time you remember. You can strain out the vanilla beans or leave them in.

Barbecue Meat Rub

Here is a flavorful meat rub you can use on many kinds of meats to be grilled, barbecued, or even roasted in the oven.

INGREDIENTS | MAKES ABOUT ½ CUP

2 tablespoons sweet paprika powder
1 tablespoon garlic powder
1 tablespoon onion powder
1 tablespoon cumin powder
½ teaspoon celery seed powder
1 teaspoon thyme leaves
1 teaspoon salt
½–1 teaspoon chili powder
½–1 teaspoon ground black pepper

Add all ingredients to an airtight jar. Use on meat by sprinkling it or rubbing it on meat before grilling, frying, or roasting. Make sure to give it a good shake before use each time to mix the flavors.

Chicken or Fish Dry Spice Rub

This meat rub is delicious on chicken or fish. You can sprinkle it onto the meat or add the spice rub to a ziplock bag, add the meat to the bag, close the bag, and then shake to coat the meat evenly. You will be giving your body a good boost of nutrition with all the spices this rub contains.

INGREDIENTS | ENOUGH FOR 4 CHICKEN THIGHS OR 4 FISH FILLETS

2 tablespoons whole coriander seed

½ teaspoon celery seed

½ teaspoon dried garlic granules

1 teaspoon dried onion granules

1 teaspoon whole peppercorns

1 teaspoon salt

¼ teaspoon dried red pepper (chili) flakes

Add all ingredients to a blender or food processor. Process until it becomes a fine powder.

Meat Preparation

Add this mixture to a plastic bag, then place meat in the bag, tie or close the bag, and shake until the meat is evenly covered. Alternatively, you can just sprinkle this mixture on meat before cooking. Then cook your meat as you would normally.

Fresh Ginger Syrup

This is a delicious way to enjoy the wonderful benefits of ginger. It has a variety of uses, including in Easy Ginger "Beer" or Ale (see Chapter 16).

INGREDIENTS | MAKES 1 CUP

1 cup fresh sliced ginger
¾ cup granulated sugar or honey
2 cups water

1. In a medium stockpot over medium-high heat, add ginger, sugar or honey, and water. Bring to a boil, reduce heat to low, and simmer 30–45 minutes or until the mixture reduces and becomes a thick syrup.

2. Strain the mixture through a sieve and pour into a glass jar. Put in the refrigerator to cool and thicken. This can be stored in the refrigerator for a few weeks or frozen in ice cube trays for much longer.

Preparation Tips

Prevent this mixture from crystallizing or cracking by making sure to brush the sides of the pot with water. You can use this syrup for making a natural ginger beer, drizzle it on cakes or ice cream, or add it to fruit punch or ice tea.

Beverages

Infusions

Herbal teas are water extractions of herbs and spices that enable the goodness of the plant part to be infused into the water. Infusions are teas that are made with the softer parts of herbs and spice. This method is used instead as these plants often contain volatile constituents that are best made with a gentler heating method that could otherwise break down or release certain constituents instead of containing them within the tea.

INGREDIENTS | MAKES 1 CUP

1 cup water
1 teaspoon spice or herb mix such as fresh ginger, cardamom seeds (crushed), peppermint leaves, rose petal, etc.

Boil water. Add your chosen spice or herb to a cup. Pour boiling water into the cup. Add a cover over the cup and leave to infuse 5–10 minutes. Take the cover off and enjoy your tea.

General Decoction

A decoction is one method to extract water-soluble nutrients and other constituents from certain medicinal plants. The decoction method works well for the "woodier" and harder parts such as barks, roots, and seeds. These parts of the plants are harder to extract by just pouring hot water over them, so the decoction is a welcome method. They require a longer preparation time than steeping and infusions of softer parts of herbs (flower tops).

INGREDIENTS | MAKES 1 CUP

1 cup water

1 teaspoon spice such as ginger, turmeric, galangal, ajowan, coriander, or fennel

1. Add water to a small saucepan along with your chosen spice.

2. Simmer covered about 20 minutes or so until the water becomes quite fragrant and takes on the color of the spice.

3. Strain out the spice and keep your aromatic decoction to drink as you please.

Ginger Tea

Ginger rhizome (root), Zingiber officinale, can be made into a delicious, warming, and tasty tea. This is great in winter to warm you up and is also great for those with inflammatory conditions such as arthritis or for women with dysmenorrhoea (period pain), due to ginger's anti-inflammatory actions.

INGREDIENTS | MAKES 2 CUPS

1 tablespoon grated fresh ginger
2 cups cold water
Honey, to taste

1. Place ginger in a small saucepan with cold water. Bring to a boil over medium-high heat. Reduce heat to low and simmer covered about 10 minutes.

2. Strain mixture into 2 teacups and serve with a bit of honey.

Fennel and Peppermint Infusion

This is a refreshing tea that is soothing to the digestive tract. This can be drunk hot or cold, and is good either way after a meal. The fennel seed and peppermint leaves are thought to help reduce bloating and flatulence.

INGREDIENTS | MAKES 2 CUPS

1 teaspoon fennel seed, crushed using a mortar and pestle
1–2 tablespoons fresh peppermint leaves, roughly torn
2 cups water or enough water to fill a teapot

1. Add fennel and peppermint to the teapot.
2. Boil water. Pour boiled water into the teapot. Leave covered to infuse for about 10 minutes.
3. Pour through a strainer into cups and enjoy.

Udaipur Ginger Chai

Chai is an integral part of Indian cuisine. Chai means "tea" in Hindi and is a combination of brewed spices and black tea (Camellia sinensis). Spices used can vary but generally may include ginger, green cardamom pods, black pepper, and cloves. It can be served with milk and sugar, and consumed regularly. This is a delicious and comforting drink, and can gently stimulate the digestive system.

INGREDIENTS | MAKES 4 SMALL CUPS

2 cups water
2 teaspoons loose-leaf black tea
½–1 cup cream or milk, or an alternative milk of your choice
2 teaspoons granulated sugar
1 tablespoon sliced fresh ginger

1. Add water to a small saucepan over medium-high heat. Bring to a boil and add tea.

2. Add milk and sugar and keep boiling.

3. While the mixture is boiling, prepare the ginger by rolling each slice with a rolling pin to crush it. Then add the ginger to the boiling tea. Keep an eye on it as it can boil over quickly. After 2–3 minutes, turn off heat.

4. Strain the mixture into small cups and enjoy your chai.

Sugar Substitutes

For this recipe, you can use granulated sugar, rapadura sugar, honey, coconut sugar, or stevia, or you can just leave the sugar out!

Rose Hot Chocolate

This recipe is a lovely way to add rose to your diet. Rose goes well with chocolate and together in this recipe they form a delicious, calming drink. You can use carob powder instead of cocoa powder if you are making this for children, as carob is caffeine-free and less stimulating than cocoa.

INGREDIENTS | MAKES 2 CUPS

1 tablespoon cocoa powder or carob powder
1 tablespoon water
2 cups full-fat or alternative milk
1–2 teaspoons sugar or honey, or less depending on taste
1 tablespoon dried rose petals

1. In a small saucepan, without turning the heat on the stove, add cocoa powder and water and mix into a paste.

2. Add milk, sugar, and rose petals. Whisk together.

3. Now heat the pan on medium-low while whisking the hot chocolate until smooth. Heat until the rose petals have softened and the mixture is fragrant, about 4–6 minutes.

4. Strain the hot chocolate and discard the rose petals.

5. Serve in mugs and enjoy this delicious and calming drink!

Chili Hot Chocolate

This recipe is inspired by ancient Mayan food cultures, as well as current-day Mexican cuisines that use cocoa and chili together.

INGREDIENTS | MAKES 1 CUP

½ cup full-fat dairy milk, or dairy-free alternative milk
½ cup water
2 small squares dark chocolate
½ stick cinnamon
⅛ teaspoon cayenne powder

1. Add milk and water to a medium saucepan and heat on medium. Add chocolate, cinnamon, and cayenne.

2. Whisk the hot chocolate and simmer about 10–15 minutes or until the chocolate melts and has combined.

3. Take out the cinnamon stick and pour the mixture into cups. Enjoy.

Masala Spice Powder

Masala chai *means "spice tea." Chai is served in Indian homes as a welcoming token for guests, as well as for everyday enjoyment. Chai is delicious all-year round; it can be made warm or hot in winter or iced in summer for a refreshing drink, especially if infused with a little bit of orange peel. To make chai you first need to make the spice mix; after that it is just a matter of boiling the tea, spices, milk, and sugar, and then straining the ingredients.*

INGREDIENTS | MAKES ABOUT ¼ CUP

5 green cardamom pods
1 stick cinnamon
3 black peppercorns
½ teaspoon fennel seed
1 bay leaf

Add cardamom, cinnamon, peppercorns, fennel, and bay leaf to a blender or mortar and pestle. Crush the masala mix until it is a rough powder. Store in a small airtight container in a dark cupboard.

Masala Chai

With Masala Chai, the longer you simmer it, the more flavorful it becomes.

INGREDIENTS | MAKES 4–6 SMALL CUPS

2½ cups water
2 teaspoons loose-leaf black tea such as Assam
2 teaspoons Masala Spice Powder (see recipe in this chapter)
1 teaspoon grated fresh ginger
½ cup full-fat or dairy-free milk
1–2 teaspoons granulated sugar or honey

1. In a medium saucepan add water and heat on medium-high until water boils. When water is boiling, add black tea. Reduce heat to low and simmer 1–2 minutes.

2. Add masala mix and ginger. Simmer until it is a nice brown color, about 3–5 minutes.

3. Add milk and sugar and simmer 2–3 minutes more.

4. Strain your chai into cups and enjoy.

Chai Variations

You can try adding a piece of fresh orange peel into the simmering chai for a burst of zesty freshness, or try adding a few fresh or dried fragrant rose petals for a hint of rose aroma. If you are a chocolate lover, try adding a few squares of dark chocolate for a chocolate chai version.

Turmeric, Apple, and Carrot Juice

This is a very refreshing and anti-inflammatory juice.

INGREDIENTS | MAKES ABOUT 1½ CUPS

1 medium carrot, cut into rounds

1 (2") piece fresh turmeric root, cut into pieces

1 medium apple, quartered

2 stalks celery, cut into small pieces

3–4 leaves peppermint

In a juicer, alternate juicing pieces of carrot, turmeric, apple, celery, and peppermint until it all has been juiced. Pour the juice into a glass and serve with a few ice cubes.

Rose, Elder Flower, and Hawthorn Tea

This is a beautiful and uplifting tea. This tea is aromatic, floral, and sweet-smelling. It is not only delicious; it is also medicinal. Rose is calming, elder flower helps with inflammation and mucus in the upper respiratory tract, and hawthorn berries are great for the cardiovascular system. This tea is nice with a bit of honey as well.

INGREDIENTS | MAKES 4 CUPS

1 tablespoon dried rose petals

1 tablespoon elder flowers

1 tablespoon hawthorn berries

4 cups water (or enough to fill your teapot)

1–2 teaspoons honey (optional)

1. Add dried ingredients to a teapot that has a strainer.

2. Boil water in a teakettle or large saucepan over medium-high heat. Once boiling, pour water in the teapot and put on the lid. Leave the tea to infuse about 10 minutes.

3. Enjoy with a bit of honey or just as it is.

Golden Milk

The benefits of drinking Golden Milk exist thanks to its main ingredient, turmeric. Turmeric is fat-soluble so it is best when eaten or drunk with a source of fat to aid in absorption. Adding a pinch of pepper is said to increase the bioavailability of turmeric as well.

INGREDIENTS | 2 LARGER CUPS OR 4 SMALLER CUPS

2 cups full-fat milk (or almond milk)

1 teaspoon freshly grated turmeric root or turmeric powder

⅛ teaspoon ground black pepper

1–2 teaspoons honey (optional)

1. Add milk, turmeric, black pepper, and honey (if using) to a medium saucepan.

2. Whisk together the mixture briskly, then turn the stove on to medium heat and cook while continuing to whisk to prevent burning. Cook 5–10 minutes.

3. Pour into mugs and enjoy.

Easy Ginger "Beer" or Ale

This method is a super-speedy way to make ginger beer and doesn't require any bacterial or yeast cultures. Ginger "beer" is a nonalcoholic soft drink/soda. This recipe does contain sugar; however, you only need a small amount of syrup for a delicious drink. Use 1–2 teaspoons of syrup per cup. This drink can be served with fresh lime slices or a teaspoon or two of lime juice for a refreshing summer drink.

INGREDIENTS | MAKES 2 CUPS

2 teaspoons Fresh Ginger Syrup (see recipe in Chapter 15), divided
2 cups carbonated water
Ice cubes
2 slices lemon or lime (optional)

1. Add 1 teaspoon syrup to each of 2 glasses.

2. Add 1 cup carbonated water to each glass and lightly stir.

3. Add a few ice cubes and a slice of lemon or lime to each.

Chrysanthemum and Goji Berry Tea

This is a very simple floral-tasting tea. You may be able to buy both goji berries and chrysanthemum from Asian grocery stores.

INGREDIENTS | MAKES 1 TEAPOT OR 4 CUPS

1 tablespoon chrysanthemum flowers
1 tablespoon dried goji berries
4 cups water or enough to fill a teapot

1. Add the flowers and berries to the teapot.

2. Boil the water in a teakettle or large saucepan and pour into the teapot. Put the lid on and leave to infuse 5–10 minutes. Strain into cups and enjoy.

CHAPTER 17

Treats, Sweets, and Snacks

Rose and Hawthorn Jellies

This recipe has some medicinal benefits as well as being
delicious. The gelatin contains glycine, which is anti-
inflammatory. Gelatin is also soothing to the gastrointestinal
tract. Rose is calming and hawthorn berries are rich in
antioxidants that are good for your cardiovascular system. Have
these homemade jellies as an occasional sweet treat. Note that
gelatin sheets/leaves come in different sizes, so follow the
directions on the packets for correct amount of liquid that can
be used.

**INGREDIENTS | MAKES 10–20 JELLIES, DEPENDING ON THE SIZE
THE JELLIES ARE CUT**

2 tablespoons gelatin powder or 4 gelatin leaves/sheets, broken up

1¾ cups water, divided

1 tablespoon dried (or fresh) hawthorn berries

4 frozen red raspberries or strawberries

1 tablespoon honey

1 teaspoon rose water

1. Add the gelatin to 1 cup water to soften for about 10 minutes.
   If using gelatin powder, sprinkle the gelatin on top of the
   water and then stir for a few seconds.

2. Meanwhile, make a decoction by adding the remaining
   water, hawthorn berries, and red berries to a medium saucepan. Turn heat to medium-high until the mixture is boiling,
   then turn heat to low and simmer with a lid on until the hawthorn berries become soft and the red berries have released
   their color into the water and the berries have become pale,
   about 10–15 minutes. The mixture may reduce, so you may
   want to add water to keep the volume of liquid at ¾ cup.

3. Strain and discard the berries. Return the liquid to the pot and simmer on low. Add honey and gelatin (discard the soaking water).

4. Simmer the mixture on very low and stir until all ingredients are dissolved, about 5 minutes. Add rose water.

5. Pour the mixture into a square glass dish that can hold about 1 cup of volume. Put the container in the refrigerator to set overnight.

6. When the jelly is set, cut into small squares and enjoy.

Delicious Variations

Once the jellies are set, you may want to dust them with powdered caster sugar (or finely ground rapadura sugar) for a "Turkish delight" look. You can also make a dark chocolate version of this recipe by dipping the jellies in melted chocolate. Place the jellies in a freezer so the chocolate hardens. When the chocolate has hardened, they are ready to eat.

Candied Ginger

Candied ginger uses honey rather than white sugar. This makes the ginger a bit more palatable. Crystallized ginger may be used to reduce nausea and motion sickness. A few pieces can be used in the short term to help reduce these symptoms. If your nausea or motion sickness persists, see your doctor.

INGREDIENTS | MAKES ABOUT 10 PIECES

¼ cup water
3–4 tablespoons honey
2" fresh ginger, sliced into bite-sized pieces

1. Add water and honey to a medium saucepan over medium-high heat. Bring to a boil, and then reduce heat to low and simmer.

2. Add gingerroot and make sure it is covered in the honey-water syrup.

3. Simmer until the mixture becomes thicker, about 10–15 minutes. You want the honey mixture to become foamy and start to "crack." The honey will start to get really sticky.

4. Once the honey is really hot and at the hard crack stage, turn off the heat. With a fork (and being very careful not to burn yourself), take each piece of honey-covered ginger out of the saucepan, tapping the ginger on the side of the pan to leave excess honey in the pan. Place the ginger pieces on nonstick baking paper. Leave the ginger to dry. (The honey should dry and harden.)

Spiced Coconut and Date "Bliss" Balls

These date and coconut balls are an easy and delicious way to incorporate a few spices into your diet. You can change up the spices to vary their flavor. They are naturally sweet due to the dates, which also help to bind the mixture together.

INGREDIENTS | MAKES ABOUT 12

1 cup dates, pitted and chopped

1 cup walnuts, almonds, or sunflower seeds

½ cup shredded coconut

1 tablespoon unsweetened cocoa powder

2 teaspoons ground cinnamon, ground ginger, or 1 teaspoon vanilla bean paste

Optional: 3–4 tablespoons shredded coconut or cocoa powder to roll the balls

1. Add dates, walnuts, almonds, or sunflower seeds, and shredded coconut to a food processor. Sprinkle the cocoa powder and chosen spice over the mixture. Process the mixture until the dates and coconut break down and the mixture binds together.

2. Roll into balls using about 2 teaspoons of the mixture for each. Optional step: roll the balls in the extra coconut or cocoa powder.

3. Leave in the refrigerator until firm and enjoy.

Persian Love Cake

Thank you to Lauren Burns, naturopath and Olympic Gold Medalist, for sharing this recipe.

INGREDIENTS | SERVES 6

8 tablespoons unsalted butter, softened, divided
13 ounces almond meal
¾ cup raw sugar
¾ packed cup brown sugar
1 teaspoon salt
2 large eggs
9 ounces Greek-style plain yogurt, plus extra to serve
1 tablespoon freshly grated nutmeg
¼ cup roughly chopped pistachios

1. Preheat the oven to 350°F. Grease a 10" springform pan with ½ tablespoon butter and line with greaseproof paper.

2. Put almond meal, sugars, salt, and remaining butter in a food processor and blend until coarse crumbs form. Spoon half of the mixture into the pan, gently pressing to cover the base evenly. Bake for 15 minutes, then remove from the oven and allow to cool slightly.

3. Add eggs, yogurt, and nutmeg to the uncooked mixture in the food processor and mix until smooth and creamy. Pour over the cooked base and smooth out with a spatula. Scatter the pistachios around the edges and bake 45–50 minutes until golden. The cake shouldn't be too soft in the middle. Give it a little jiggle—if the middle moves, return it to the oven for a little longer.

4. Let the cake cool in the tin for 10 minutes, and then run a knife around the edges of the tin if needed and release the springform clasp. Serve at room temperature with extra yogurt. The cake can be stored in an airtight container for up to 1 week.

Note on Nutmeg

Even though a whole nutmeg is used in this recipe, don't be deterred. It is distributed evenly in the cake.

Rice Pudding

This creamy Rice Pudding is flavored with lemon zest and cardamom. You can also add 1 tablespoon of rose petals when boiling the milk to add a nice floral flavor to the pudding.

INGREDIENTS | SERVES 4–6

1 cup uncooked basmati rice
2 cups water
2½ cups full-fat milk (or alternative milk)
2 cardamom pods, crushed
1 teaspoon lemon zest
¼ cup granulated or raw sugar
1 teaspoon vanilla extract
¼ cup raisins
Grated nutmeg for garnish
¼ cup roughly chopped pistachios

1. In a large saucepan, boil the uncooked rice in 2 cups water in a pot at medium heat until very soft, about 20–30 minutes (or just use 1 cup of leftover cooked basmati rice and add 1 cup of water, which you will use in the next step). When cooked, strain off about half of the water.

2. Add milk, cardamom, lemon zest, sugar, vanilla extract, and raisins to the cooked rice.

3. Simmer this mixture over very low heat, stirring continuously, until it becomes thick and creamy, about 20–30 minutes. You may need to add more milk or water if the mixture gets too thick.

4. Serve garnished with grated nutmeg and chopped pistachios.

CHAPTER 18

The Spice Apothecary

Black Pepper–Infused Oil

This body oil is for external use. It can be used to massage into sore and tired muscles. A small amount can even be used on the scalp as a stimulating massage oil.

INGREDIENTS | MAKES ABOUT 1 CUP

½ cup whole black peppercorns
1 cup olive oil, almond oil, or sesame oil

1. Add black peppercorns to a blender or coffee grinder and roughly grind the peppercorns until coarse (not fine).

2. Add ground peppercorns to a glass jar and stir in the oil.

3. Put the lid on tightly and give the oil a good shake. Label the jar with the date and what is in the jar then leave to infuse. Give the jar a shake every day and leave to infuse for 2 weeks.

Infused Oils

Infused oils can be made in small or large quantities. When making infused oils always use dried rather than fresh herbs to prevent the growth of mold. This recipe can be made fairly quickly in a dehydrator, or a bit slower, but still effectively, by hand as a cold-infused oil.

Warming Black Pepper and Cinnamon Salve

A salve is a waxy emulsion of oil and beeswax that is solid at room temperature. It absorbs easily into the skin. This recipe makes a nice warming salve to use on sore, tired muscles. You can also use a little of this on dry scalps.

INGREDIENTS | MAKES ½ CUP

½ cup Black Pepper–Infused Oil (see recipe in this chapter)
1 tablespoon grated or chopped beeswax
2 drops *Cinnamom vernum* essential oil
3–4 drops vitamin E oil

1. In a large saucepan, simmer 3 inches of water over low heat and place a medium-sized stainless steel bowl in the pot, making sure it is snug and won't move around.

2. Put oil in the stainless steel bowl along with beeswax. Stir and heat the oil until the beeswax has melted.

3. Add cinnamon and vitamin E oils. Stir 3–4 minutes longer.

4. Pour the mixture into a tin or glass jar. Allow to firm at room temperature. Use as needed, about a pea-sized amount on the skin over sore muscles.

Salve Safety

It is important that you do not use this salve on broken skin and do not ingest it either. It is for external use only.

Geraldine's Winter Syrup and Cordial

Thank you to naturopath Geraldine Headley (and her mother Patricia) for sharing this recipe. This syrup recipe is a cordial, which may help to ward off colds and flus. You can use it hot or cold. For example, you can add 1–2 teaspoons to some hot water for a tea or add 1–2 teaspoons to cold water for a refreshing drink.

INGREDIENTS | MAKES 3 CUPS

1 cup lemon or lime juice
Rind of 2 lemons (or 3 limes)
2 cups coconut sugar
1 cup manuka honey
1 tablespoon tartaric acid
1 tablespoon citric acid
1 tablespoon Epsom salts (magnesium sulfate)
5 cups water
1 cup elder flowers
1 cup rose hips

1. Place lemon juice and rind in a medium bowl with the sugar, honey, acids, and salt, stirring occasionally for 5 minutes.

2. Boil water with the elder flowers and rose hips in a large saucepan over medium-high heat. Once boiling, reduce heat to low and simmer 30 minutes. You need 3 cups by the end of cooking, so you may need to add more water occasionally if it looks like it is boiling dry.

3. Strain out the bits and add honey mixture, stirring until all the sugar is dissolved. Cover and allow to cool to room temperature.

4. Strain out the rinds, pour into a bottle or other container, and store in the refrigerator.

Flower Power

If you don't have elder flowers, don't worry. You can leave them out of this recipe. The lemon cordial with honey is delicious enough on its own.

Honey and Onion Cough Syrup

This is a nice cough syrup for colds and flus. It helps to break down mucus in the respiratory tract. You should avoid using raw honey if you are making this for children. You should also avoid this if you are allergic to honey and other bee products or onions.

INGREDIENTS | MAKES ABOUT ½ CUP SYRUP

1 medium brown onion, peeled and finely chopped
1 tablespoon honey

1. Add onion to a small bowl and add honey. Stir together.

2. Put a piece of cling wrap over the bowl.

3. Place the bowl in the refrigerator and leave for a few hours. During this process, the honey will extract the juice from the onion and it will form a syrup.

4. When quite a bit of the liquid has been drawn out of the honey, strain the mixture and discard the onion. Keep leftover syrup in a lidded contain in the refrigerator for 1–2 days, after which you should discard it.

Thyme-Infused Honey

You can use this Thyme-Infused Honey to soothe sore throats. Thyme is a wonderful herb for the upper respiratory system. This herbal honey can be added to herbal teas or eaten off a spoon when you have a sore throat or cough due to the common cold or flu.

INGREDIENTS | MAKES 1 CUP

½ cup dried thyme leaves
1 cup honey

1. Add thyme leaves to a jar. Add honey and mix together.

2. Label it with the date and what it is. Leave in a sunny or warm spot to infuse 2–3 weeks. Give it a stir or a shake every few days.

3. Strain the herbs out of the honey and keep the honey in the glass jar. To strain the herbs out of the honey, gently heat the jar containing the infused honey in a saucepan with a few inches of water. Warm the honey until it becomes pourable. Turn off the heat and discard the water in the pot. Pour this honey through a fine strainer until all the dried herbs have been filtered out. Alternatively you can just leave the thyme leaves in the honey.

Important Note

Only used dried thyme leaves in this recipe. Fresh leaves, due to their water content, carry a risk of bacterial growth. You can make a similar honey with dried rose petals or sage leaves.

Licorice and Cucumber Face Scrub

In this face scrub recipe, the licorice and cucumber are soothing due to licorice's emollient actions and cucumber's cooling attributes. This face scrub will make your face feel very soft due to the mucilaginous content of the licorice. This recipe is to be used topically on the skin.

INGREDIENTS | MAKES ENOUGH FACE SCRUB FOR 2 PEOPLE

1 tablespoon finely ground dried licorice root
2 tablespoons finely grated fresh cucumber

1. In a small bowl, mix together licorice and cucumber until you have a smooth paste.

2. Apply the mixture to your face and use a circular motion to gently scrub your skin for a few minutes, avoiding your eyes.

3. Wash off the face mask (you can put it in the compost or the garden) and then moisturize as per your usual routine.

Namak (Salt) and Adrak (Ginger)

Namak *means "salt" and* adrak *means "ginger" in Hindi. This is a very simple home remedy that is effective when you have a cold or the flu. Those with hypertension or who have been told to reduce salt intake should avoid this recipe.*

INGREDIENTS | MAKES 1 TABLESPOON

2 tablespoons chopped fresh ginger
½ tablespoon sea salt

1. In a small sauté pan, dry roast the ginger over medium-high heat 3–5 minutes. Add salt. Dry roast another 3–5 minutes.

2. Remove ginger from pan and let cool. You can chew a few small pieces when suffering with a cold or flu. They can be stored in a sealed container for a few days in the fridge.

Sage and Mint Mouthwash

This is a simple and inexpensive mouthwash recipe that will freshen your breath naturally.

INGREDIENTS | MAKES 1 CUP

1 cup water
1 teaspoon chopped fresh sage leaves
1 teaspoon chopped fresh mint leaves

1. In a small saucepan, boil water over medium-high heat, and then turn off the heat once boiled. Add sage and mint and leave to infuse, with a lid on, about 10 minutes. Let cool completely.

2. When cool, use as a mouthwash by swishing a mouthful or so in your mouth. Discard after 1 day.

Rosemary Tonic Hair Rinse

Rosemary and apple cider vinegar are great ingredients for the health of the hair and the scalp. Rosemary is antimicrobial, which can help reduce dandruff, and it is also thought to stimulate hair growth, especially when it is massaged onto the scalp.

INGREDIENTS | MAKES 1 CUP

1 cup apple cider vinegar
½ cup chopped fresh rosemary leaves

1. Pour apple cider vinegar into a glass jar. Add rosemary to a jar and then screw the lid on tight to seal the jar.

2. Label the jar with the contents and the date. Give the jar a shake every day to help infuse the rosemary into the vinegar.

3. After 2 weeks, strain out rosemary leaves and store vinegar mixture in a spray bottle.

4. Apply 1 tablespoon to your head and massage into your scalp after showers.

Rose and Almond Body Oil

This a wonderful, aromatic rose body oil. The rose petals not only make it smell floral but they also add their own unique antibacterial benefits to the oil.

INGREDIENTS | MAKES 1 CUP

1 cup sweet almond oil, olive oil, or coconut oil
1 cup dried rose petals

1. Add oil and rose petals to a glass jar and screw on lid. Give the glass jar a good shake to evenly mix together the oil and the rose petals.

2. Shake the oil every day or as often as you remember for 2–4 weeks.

3. Leave the oil in a cool, dark place such as in the back of a pantry cupboard to help extract the rose into the oil and to prevent the oil from oxidizing.

4. After 2–4 weeks, strain out the rose. You can store the oil in the glass container and using a clean dry spoon, scoop some of the oil out as you need it, making sure to close the jar tightly after each use.

Points to Consider

This oil can be used on your face or body. You can also keep the rose petals and mix them with a bit of sugar for a nice body scrub. You can try making this with coconut oil in warmer seasons. It is important to use dried rose petals rather than fresh to avoid any bacteria growth in the finished product. You can add a few teaspoons of this oil in the bath, along with some full-fat milk, for a luxurious and relaxing bath.

Glossary

Herbal Actions Used in Western Herbal Medicine

Plants, herbs, and spices offer you many benefits for your health and well-being. Following are some of the actions mentioned in this book. You will also find the definitions of important words pertinent to spices and health used throughout the text.

Adaptive immunity
Also known as the acquired immune system. It is developed over time and life by learning and adapting to pathogens.

Adrenal glands
Endocrine glands located above each kidney. The adrenal glands are responsible for secreting steroid hormones and epinephrine and norepinephrine.

Adrenaline
A hormone excreted by the adrenal glands in times of stress.

Aerial parts
The parts of a plant that grow above the ground and include leaves, flowers, and stems.

Analgesic
Analgesic substances have pain-relieving properties or help to reduce pain.

Antibacterial
Antibacterial herbs help to interfere with microbes and bacteria.

Anti-emetic
Anti-emetics help reduce the feeling of nausea and reduce or prevent vomiting.

Anti-inflammatory
Anti-inflammatory herbs help reduce inflammation in the body.

Antioxidant
An antioxidant is a substance that reduces oxidation in the body or reduces free radical damage.

Antispasmodic
Antispasmodic herbs help reduce spasms of smooth-muscle fiber tissues in the body.

Antiviral
Antiviral herbs help prevent viruses from proliferating or reduce viral infections.

Aromatherapy
The practice of inhaling essential oils from flowers, plants, barks, etc., to increase health and well-being.

Astringent
Astringent herbs usually contain tannins, which constrict the internal mucous membranes. They create a "puckering" feeling in

the mouth and tongue due to tannin content, which interacts with proteins.

Atherosclerosis
Coronary artery atherosclerosis is the main cause of cardiovascular disease. In coronary artery atherosclerosis, the walls of the coronary arteries become damaged due to fat deposits in the inner artery walls.

Ayurveda
The main traditional medicine system in India. The word *Ayurveda* can be translated to mean "the Science of Life." Ayurveda combines the use of herbal medicine, yoga, and dietary therapies.

Bitter
Bitter-tasting herbs are usually used to stimulate poor digestion.

Botany
The scientific study of plants.

Carminative
A carminative is a substance that helps calm and reduce gas and flatulence in the digestive system.

Circulatory stimulant
A circulatory stimulant helps to encourage healthy blood circulation in the body.

Complementary and alternative medicine (CAM)
In CAM, herbs and spices are used as a part of your diet for medicinal purposes. The main forms of CAM include nutritional and herbal products, as well as massage, acupuncture, naturopathy, and yoga.

Cortisol
A hormone released by your adrenal glands. It mobilizes and stimulates the production of substances such as protein and glucose to be used by the body in times of stress.

Demulcent
Demulcent herbs contain mucilage, which acts to soothe and reduce inflammation of the body's mucosa.

Emollient
An emollient herb is similar to a demulcent in that it soothes tissues; however, they are generally topically applied to the skin.

Enzymes
A substance produced by a living organism that prompts a biochemical reaction.

Epinephrine
Epinephrine is a hormone used by the body in the "fight or flight" response. This hormone affects cardiac function by increasing the heart's contractions. It also increases heart rate and blood pressure, and it dilates the blood vessels, causing greater blood flow to the muscles. It also increases blood sugar levels.

Epithelial cells
Layer of cells that line hollow organs or glands.

Expectorants
An expectorant is an herb that helps the body expel mucus from the respiratory tract.

Gastric acid
Digestive fluid found in the stomach.

Gut microbiota
A complex mix of microorganisms found in the digestive tract.

Hepatoprotective
Hepatoprotective herbs help protect and reduce damage in the liver.

Herbal medicine
The science and art of using plants and herbal medicines to improve health and well-being.

Hypocholesterolemic
Hypocholesterolemic herbs help reduce cholesterol levels.

Hypotensive
Hypotensive herbs are thought to aid in a reduction of blood pressure.

Immunoglobulins
Also known as antibodies, they are an important part of your immune system, as they bind to bacteria or viruses to help destroy them.

Innate immune system
The first line of defense against foreign bodies such as bacteria, toxins, and viruses. It includes physical barriers such as the skin, mucous membranes, and processes such as inflammation.

Magnesium
A mineral that has hundreds of functions in the body including metabolizing energy, glucose control, and regulating blood pressure.

Metabolism
A biological process in the body that converts food into energy.

Microbe
A microorganism.

Mucolytic
Mucolytic herbs help break down excess mucus.

Naturopathy
A system that combines the use of herbal medicine, dietary therapies, nutritional medicine, massage, and lifestyle adjustments.

Nootropic
A nootropic is a substance that stimulates the brain and cognition, and improves memory.

Oxidation
A chemical process that causes damage to body cells due to an imbalance of free radicals and antioxidants.

Pepsin
Enzyme in the stomach that breaks down proteins.

Phagocytes
Cells in the body that engulf bacteria and other particles.

Serotonin
A neurotransmitter known as the "happy" hormone. It regulates mood, social behavior, appetite, and other functions such as digestion.

Sialagogue
A sialagogue is a substance that stimulates saliva production.

Spasmolytic

A spasmolytic herb is one that helps reduce spasms in skeletal muscle.

Synergy

In herbal medicine, synergy refers to the interaction of two or more herbs (or substances) that complement the actions of each herbal medicine.

Traditional Chinese medicine

Includes therapies such as acupuncture (including cupping, moxibustion, and Qi Gong, which is similar to tai chi), herbal medicine, dietary therapies, lifestyle therapies, and a type of massage called tui na.

Vitamin B_{12}

A crucial water-soluble vitamin needed for nerve health, metabolism, and for the production of red blood cells that carry oxygen throughout the body.

Vitamin D

A fat-soluble vitamin that is essential for the absorption of calcium.

Western herbal medicine (WHM)

WHM uses a combination of long-established (traditional), current, and up-to-date evidence-based information in the therapeutic prescription of herbal medicine to improve health and well-being.

APPENDIX B

Further Reading and Bibliography

Adams, J., and E. Tan. *Herbal Manufacturing: How to Make Medicines from Plants* (Melbourne: Adams and Tan, 2006).

Bitcon, C. "Seven Herbs for the Modern Woman Series: Rose." (2014) *http://elmbotanicals.blogspot.com/2014/05/seven-herbs-for-modern-woman-series-rose.html*, accessed July 2015.

Braun, L., and Cohen, M. *Herbs and Natural Supplements: An Evidence-Based Guide*, 3rd Edition (Elsevier, Australia: Churchill Livingstone, 2010).

Culpeper, N. *Culpeper's Complete Herbal* (London: Richard Evans, 1816).

Duke, J. *CRC Handbook of Medicinal Spices* (Boca Raton, FL: CRC Press, 2003).

Duke, J. *Dr. Duke's Phytochemical and Ethnobotanical Databases*, *www.ars-grin.gov/duke*, accessed June 2015.

Ellingwood, F. *American Materia Medica, Therapeutics and Pharmacognosy* (Bisbee, AZ: Southwest School of Botanical Medicine, 1919).

Gladstar, R. *Rosemary Gladstar's Medicinal Herbs: A Beginner's Guide* (North Adams, MA: Storey Publishing, 2012).

Hechtman, L. *Clinical Naturopathic Medicine* (Elsevier, Australia: Churchill Livingstone, 2012).

Heinrich, M., et al. *Fundamentals of Pharmacognosy and Phytotherapy* (Elsevier, Australia: Churchill Livingstone, 2004).

Hoffman, D. *Holistic Herbal: A Safe and Practical Guide to Making and Using Herbal Remedies* (London: Thorsons, 2004).

Khare, C.P. *Indian Medicinal Plants: An Illustrated Dictionary* (Berlin, Germany: Springer Science & Business Media, 2008).

McCance, K.L., and Huether, S.E. *Pathophysiology: The Biologic Basis for Disease in Adults and Children* (Missouri: Mosby Elsevier, 2010).

McGee, H. *On Food and Cooking: The Science and Lore of the Kitchen* (New York: Fireside, 1984).

Moore, M. *Herbal Materia Medica*, 5th Edition (Bisbee, AZ: Southwest School of Botanical Medicine, 1995), *www.swsbm.com/ManualsMM/MatMed5.pdf*, accessed June 2015.

Moore. M. *An Herbal/Medical Dictionary* (Bisbee, AZ: Southwest School of Botanical Medicine, 1995), *www.swsbm.com/ManualsMM/MedHerbGloss2.pdf*, accessed September 2015.

Moore, M. *Principles and Practice of Constitutional Physiology for Herbalists* (Bisbee, AZ: Southwest School of Botanical Medicine, 1985).

Priest, A.W., and Priest, L.R. *Herbal Medication: A Clinical and Dispensary Handbook* (London: L.N. Fowler & Co., 1982).

Ravindran, P.N., and Madhusoodanan, K.J. *Cardamom: The Genus Elettaria* (London: CRC Press, 2002).

Rose, K. "Wild Rose Elixir: A Favorite First Aid Remedy." *The Medicine Woman's Roots*, (2008), *http://bearmedicineherbals.com/wild-rose-elixir-a-favorite-first-aid-remedy.html*, accessed July 2015.

Turner, J. *Spice: The History of a Temptation* (New York: A.A. Knopf, 2004).

United States Pharmacopedial Convention. *The Pharmacopeia of the United States of America*, 8th Decennial Revision (New York: P. Blakiston's Son & Company, 1900).

Wood, M. *The Earthwise Herbal: A Complete Guide to Old World Medicinal Plants* (Berkeley, CA: North Atlantic Books, 2008).

Studies on Spices and Supporting Information

Ben-Yehoshua, S. "Frankincense, Myrrh, and Balm of Gilead: Ancient Spices." *Horticultural Reviews*, 39 (2012).

Carding, S., Verbeke, K., Vipond, D.T., Corfe, B.M., and Owen, L.J. "Dysbiosis of the Gut Microbiota in Disease." *Microbial Ecology in Health and Disease*, 26 (2015), *www.microbecolhealthdis.net/index.php/mehd/article/view/26191*, accessed September 2015.

CPMCNET. Michael D. Gershon, MD, Department of Anatomy and Cell Biology. (2001), *www.cumc.columbia.edu/dept/gsas/anatomy/Faculty/Gershon*, accessed September 2015.

Darling, L.M. *History of Spice Trade*. UCLA Biomedical Library, History & Special Collections (2002), *https://unitproj.library.ucla.edu/biomed/spice/index.cfm?spicefilename=TimelineHistorySpiceTrade.txt&itemsuppress=yes&displayswitch=0*, accessed September 2015.

Eknoyan, G. "Armenian Medicine and Diseases of the Kidney." *Journal of Nephrology*, 22 (2009), *www.ncbi.nlm.nih.gov/pubmed/20013725*, accessed July 2015.

Ersnt, E. "Frankincense: Systematic Review." *British Medical Journal*, 337:a2813 (2008), *www.ncbi.nlm.nih.gov/pmc/articles/PMC2605614/pdf/bmj.a2813.pdf.*

Fan, J.G., and Cao, H.X. "Role of Diet and Nutritional Management in Non-alcoholic Fatty Liver Disease." *Journal of Gastroenterology and Hepatology*, 28(4) (2013), *www.ncbi.nlm.nih.gov/pubmed/24251710*, accessed September 2015.

Farjana, H.N., Chandrasekaran, S.C., and Gita, B. "Effect of Oral Curcuma Gel in Gingivitis Management: A Pilot Study." *Journal of Clinical and Diagnostic Research*, 8(12) (2014).

Hausenblas, H.A., et al. "Saffron (*Crocus sativus L.*) and Major Depressive Disorder: A Meta-analysis of Randomized Clinical Trials." *Journal of Integrative Medicine*, 11(6) (2013), *www.jcimjournal.com/jim/FullText2.aspx?articleID=jintegrmed2013056*, accessed June 2015.

Hodges, R.E., and Minich, D.M. "Modulation of Metabolic Detoxification Pathways Using Foods and Food-Derived Components: A Scientific Review with Clinical Application." *Journal of Nutrition and Metabolism*, 2015 (2015), *www.hindawi.com/journals/jnme/2015/760689*, accessed September 2015.

Hosseinzadeh, H., and Younesi, H.M. "Antinociceptive and Anti-inflammatory Effects of *Crocus sativus L.* Stigma and Petal Extracts in Mice." *BMC Pharmacology*, 2(7) (2002), *www.biomedcentral.com/1471-2210/2/7*, accessed June 2015.

Hu, M.L., et al. "Effect of Ginger on Gastric Motility and Symptoms of Functional Dyspepsia." *World Journal of*

Gastroenterology, 17(1) (2011), *www.ncbi.nlm.nih.gov/pmc/articles/PMC3016669*, accessed June 2015.

Hursel, R., Viechtbauer, W., and Westerterp-Plantenga, M.S. "The Effects of Green Tea on Weight Loss and Weight Maintenance: A Meta-analysis." *International Journal of Obesity*, 22 (2009), *www.nature.com/ijo/journal/v33/n9/full/ijo2009135a.html*, accessed September 2015.

Ibrahim, R.M., Hamdan, N.S., Ismail, M., Saini, S.M., Abd Rashid, S.N., Abd Latiff, L., and Mahmud, R. "Protective Effects of *Nigella sativa* on Metabolic Syndrome in Menopausal Women." *Advanced Pharmaceutical Bulletin*, 4(1) (2014), *www.ncbi.nlm.nih.gov/pmc/articles/PMC3885365*, accessed September 2015.

Igarashi, M., et al. "Effect of Olfactory Simulation by Fresh Rose Flowers on Autonomic Nervous Activity." *Journal of Alternative and Complementary Medicine*, 20(9) (2014), *www.ncbi.nlm.nih.gov/pubmed/25055057*, accessed May 2015.

Iluz, D., et al. "Medicinal Properties of *Commiphora gileadensis*." *African Journal of Pharmacy and Pharmacology*, 4(8) (2010).

Jankasem, M., Wuthi-udomlert, M., Gritsanapan, W. "Antidermatophytic Properties of Ar-Turmerone, Turmeric Oil, and Curcuma longa Preparations." *ISRN Dermatology*, 2013 (2013), *www.hindawi.com/journals/isrn/2013/250597/cta*, accessed September 2015.

Josse, A.R., Sherriffs, S.S., Holwerda, A.M., Andrews, R., Staples, A.W., and Phillips, S.M. "Effects of Capsinoid Ingestion on Energy Expenditure and Lipid Oxidation at Rest and During Exercise." *Nutrition & Metabolism*, 7(65) (2010), *www.nutritionandmetabolism.com/content/7/1/65*, accessed July 2015.

Khodaie, L., and Sadeghpoor, O. "Ginger from Ancient Times to the New Outlook." *Jundishapur Journal of Natural Pharmaceutical Products*, 10(1) (2015), *www.ncbi.nlm.nih.gov/pmc/articles/pmid/25866718*, accessed June 2015.

Latel, K., and Srinivasan, K. "Digestive Stimulant Action of Spices: A Myth or Reality?" *Indian Journal of Medical Research*, 119(5) (2004), *www.ncbi.nlm.nih.gov/pubmed/15218978*, accessed June 2015.

Latiff, L.A., Parhizkar, S., Dollah, M.A., and Hassan, S.T.S. "Alternative Supplement for Enhancement of Reproductive Health and Metabolic Profile Among Perimenopausal Women: A Novel Role of *Nigella sativa*." *Iranian Journal of Basic Medical Sciences*, 17(12) (2014), *www.ncbi.nlm.nih.gov/pmc/articles/PMC4387233*, accessed September 2015.

Leise, M.D., Poterucha, J.J., and Talwalkar, J.A. "Drug-Induced Liver Injury." *Mayo Clinic Proceedings*, 89(1) (2014), *www.ncbi.nlm.nih.gov/pubmed/24388027*, accessed September 2015.

Liska, D.J. "The Detoxification Enzyme Systems." *Alternative Medicine Review*, 3(3) (1998), *www.altmedrev.com/publications/3/3/187.pdf*, accessed September 2015.

Lontchi-Yimagou, E., Sobngwi, E., Matsha, T.E., and Kengne, A.P. "Diabetes Mellitus and Inflammation." *Diabetes and Other Diseases–Emerging Associations, Current Diabetes Reports*, 13(3) (2013).

Mahendra, P., and Bisht, S. "Ferula Asafoetida: Traditional Uses and Pharmacological Activity." *Pharmacognosy Reviews*, 6(12) (2012), *www.ncbi.nlm.nih.gov/pmc/articles/PMC3459456*, accessed June 2015.

Mansour, G., et al. "Clinical Efficacy of New Aloe Vera- and Myrrh-Based Oral Mucoadhesive Gels in the Management of Minor Recurrent Aphthous Stomatitis: A Randomized, Double-Blind, Vehicle-Controlled Study." *Journal of Oral Pathology and Medicine*, 43(6) (2014), *www.ncbi.nlm.nih .gov/pubmed/24164309*, accessed June 2015.

Mastroiacovo, D., Kwik-Uribe, C., Grassi, D., Necozione, S., et al. "Cocoa Flavanol Consumption Improves Cognitive Function, Blood Pressure Control, and Metabolic Profile in Elderly Subjects: The Cocoa, Cognition, and Aging (CoCoA) Study; A Randomized Controlled Trial." *American Journal of Clinical Nutrition*, 101(3) (2015), *www.ncbi .nlm.nih.gov/pmc/articles/PMC4340060*, accessed June 2015.

Mehmood, M.H., and Gilani, A.H. "Pharmacological Basis for the Medicinal Use of Black Pepper and Piperine in Gastrointestinal Disorders." *Journal of Medicinal Food*, 13(5) (2010), *www.ncbi.nlm.nih.gov/pubmed/20828313*, accessed June 2015.

Murlidhar, M., and Goswami, T.K. "Nutritional Constituent of Black Pepper as Medicinal Molecules: A Review." *Open Access Scientific Reports*, 1(1) (2012).

Nagpal, M., and Sood, S. "Role of Curcumin in Systemic and Oral Health: An Overview." *Journal of Natural Science, Biology and Medicine*, 4 (2013), *www.jnsbm.org/text .asp?2013/4/1/3/107253*, accessed June 2015.

National Cancer Institute. "Chronic Inflammation." National Institute of Health (2015), *www.cancer.gov/about-cancer/ causes-prevention/risk/chronic-inflammation*, accessed September 2015.

Nobre, A.C., Rao, A., and Owen, G.N. "L-theanine, a Natural Constituent in Tea, and Its Effect on Mental State." *Asia Pacific Journal of Clinical Nutrition*, 17(1) (2008).

Percival, M. "Phytonutrients & Detoxification." *Clinical Nutrition Insights*, 5(2), (1997), *www.acudoc.com/phytonutrientsand detoxification.PDF*, accessed September 2015.

Platel, K., and Srinivasan, K. "Digestive Stimulant Action of Spices: A Myth or Reality?" *The Indian Journal of Medical Research*, 119(5) (2004), *www.ncbi.nlm.nih.gov/pubmed/15218978*, accessed August 2015.

Poirier, P., Giles, T.D., Bray, G.A., Hong, Y., Stern, J.S., Pi-Sunyer, X., and Eckel, R.H. "Obesity and Cardiovascular Disease: Pathophysiology, Evaluation, and Effect of Weight Loss." *Circulation*, 2006(113) (2006), *http://circ.ahajournals.org/content/113/6/898.full*, accessed September 2015.

Puram, S., et al. "Effect of GutGard in the Management of *Helicobacter pylori*: A Randomized Double Blind Placebo Controlled Study." *Evidence-Based Complementary and Alternative Medicine*, 2013 (2013), *www.ncbi.nlm.nih.gov/pmc/articles/PMC3623263*, accessed June 2015.

Rajsekhar, S., and Kuldeep, B. "Pharmacognosy and Pharmacology of *Nigella sativa*: A Review." *International Research Journal of Pharmacy*, 2(11) (2011), *www.irjponline.com/admin/php/uploads/673_pdf.pdf*, accessed September 2015.

Ramos-Nino, M.E. "The Role of Chronic Inflammation in Obesity-Associated Cancers." *ISRN Oncology*, 2013 (2013).

Rao, P.S., et al. "An Important Spice, *Pimenta dioica* (Linn.) Merill: A Review." *International Current Pharmaceutical Journal*, 1(8) (2012), *www.icpjonline.com/documents/Vol1Issue8/08.pdf*.

Rašković, A., Milanović, I., Pavlović, N., Ćebović, T., Vukmirović, S., and Mikov, M. "Antioxidant Activity of Rosemary (*Rosmarinus officinalis* (L.) Essential Oil and Its Hepatoprotective Potential." *BMC Complementary and Alternative Medicine*, 14(225) (2014), *www.ncbi.nlm.nih.gov/pmc/articles/PMC4227022*, accessed May 2015.

Ried, K., and Fakler, P. "Potential of Garlic (*Allium sativum*) in Lowering High Blood Pressure: Mechanisms of Action and Clinical Relevance." *Integrated Blood Pressure Control*, 9(7) (2014), *www.ncbi.nlm.nih.gov/pmc/articles/PMC4266250*, accessed June 2015.

Saenghong, N., et al. "*Zingiber officinale* Improves Cognitive Function of the Middle-Aged Healthy Women." *Evidence-Based Complementary and Alternative Medicine*, 2012 (2012), *www.hindawi.com/journals/ecam/2012/383062*.

Sahoo, H.B., Sahoo, S.K., Sarangi, S.P., Sagar, R., and Kori, M.L. "Anti-diarrhoeal Investigation from Aqueous Extract of *Cuminum cyminum Linn.* Seed in Albino Rats." *Pharmacognosy Research*, 6(3) (2014), *www.ncbi.nlm.nih.gov/pmc/articles/PMC4080500*, accessed June 2015.

Schneider, R.H., Grim, C.E., Rainforth, M.V., Kotchen, T., Nidich, S.I., Gaylord-King, C., Salerno, J.W., Kotchen, J.M., and Alexander, C.N. "Stress Reduction in the Secondary Prevention of Cardiovascular Disease: Randomized, Controlled Trial of Transcendental Meditation and Health Education in Blacks." *Circulation: Cardiovascular Quality and Outcomes*, (2012), *http://circoutcomes.ahajournals.org/content/early/2012/11/13/CIRCOUTCOMES.112.967406*, accessed September 2015.

Selye, H. "Stress and the General Adaptation Syndrome." *British Medical Journal*, 1(4667), (1950), *www.ncbi.nlm.nih.gov/pmc/articles/PMC2038162*, accessed September 2015.

Shabbir, A. "*Rhus coriaria* Linn, a Plant of Medicinal, Nutritional and Industrial Importance: A Review." *Journal of Animal and Plant Sciences*, 22(2) (2012), *www.researchgate.net/publication/233860365_Rhus_coriaria_Linn_a_plant_of_medicinal_nutritional_and_industrial_importance_A_review*, accessed September 2015.

Siddiqui, M.Z. "*Boswellia serrata*, a Potential Antiinflammatory Agent: An Overview." *Indian Journal of Pharmaceutical Sciences*, 73(3) (2011), *www.ijpsonline.com/text.asp?2011/73/3/255/93507*, accessed September 2015.

Slavich, G.M., and Irwin, M.R. "From Stress to Inflammation and Major Depressive Disorder: A Social Signal Transduction Theory of Depression." *Psychological Bulletin*, 140(3) (2014), *http://dx.doi.org/10.1037/a0035302*, accessed August 2015.

Snitker, S., Fujishima, Y., Shen, H., Ott, S., Pi-Sunyer, X., Furuhata, Y., Sato, H., and Takahashi, M. "Effects of Novel Capsinoid Treatment on Fatness and Energy Metabolism in Humans: Possible Pharmacogenetic Implications." *American Society for Nutrition*, 89(1) (2008), *http://ajcn.nutrition.org/content/89/1/45.full*, accessed July 2015.

Srinivasan, K. "Black Pepper and Its Pungent Principle-Piperine: A Review of Diverse Physiological Effects." *Critical Reviews in Food and Science Nutrition*, 47(8) (2007), *www.ncbi.nlm.nih.gov/pubmed/17987447*, accessed August 2015.

Thompson, A., Meah, D., Ahmed, N., Conniff-Jenkins, R., Chileshe, E., Phillips, C.O., Claypole, T.C., Forman, D.W., and Row, P.E. "Comparison of the Antibacterial Activity of Essential Oils and Extracts of Medicinal and Culinary Herbs to Investigate Potential New Treatments for Irritable Bowel Syndrome." *BMC Complementary and Alternative Medicine*, 28(12, 228) (2013), *www.ncbi.nlm.nih.gov/pubmed/24283351*, accessed August 2015.

White, B. "Ginger: An Overview." *American Family Physician*, 1(75, 11) (2007), *www.aafp.org/afp/2007/0601/p1689.html*, accessed June 2015.

Wing, R.R., Lang, W., Wadden, T.A., Safford, M., Knowler, W.C., et al. "Benefits of Modest Weight Loss in Improving Cardiovascular Risk Factors in Overweight and Obese Individuals With Type 2 Diabetes." *Diabetes Care*, 34 (2011), *http://care.diabetesjournal.org/content/34/7/1481.full*, accessed September 2015.

Yoto, A., et al. "Effects of L-theanine or Caffeine Intake on Changes in Blood Pressure Under Physical and Psychological Stresses." *Journal of Physiological Anthropology*, 31(1, 28) (2012), *www.ncbi.nlm.nih.gov/pmc/articles/PMC3518171*, accessed July 2015.

Youssef, H., and Mousa, R. "Nutritional Assessment of Low-Calorie Baladi Rose Petals Jam." *Food and Public Health*, 2(6) (2012), *http://article.sapub.org/10.5923.j.fph.20120206.03.html*, accessed July 2015.

APPENDIX C

Table of Spices

SPICES AND POPULAR USE

Spice	Use
Ajowan	Used as a digestion-improving spice and as a remedy to combat an upset stomach.
Allspice	Used for digestive complaints, as an aphrodisiac, as an anodyne, and for nerve pain (neuralgia).
Aniseed	Used as an expectorant, as a digestive tonic, to relieve heartburn, as an emmenagogue (herbs that stimulate blood flow in the pelvic area and uterus), a galactagogue (stimulates flow of mother's breast milk), and an aphrodisiac.
Asafetida	Used as a stimulating expectorant, antispasmodic (reduces spasms), carminative, laxative, sedative, vermifuge, diuretic, anthelmintic (herbs that expel parasitic worms), an aphrodisiac, and an emmenagogue.
Bay Leaf	Has antioxidant properties and has been used to treat digestive issues.
Black Pepper	Used for its digestive properties such as antispasmodic, carminative (herbs that prevent or treat excess gas), digestive stimulant, and possible antidiarrheal. It is also a good herb for the immune system when used as an expectorant.
Calendula	Reduces inflammation as an anti-inflammatory flower, and is also antibacterial, lymphatic, and a wound healer.
Caraway	Used to soothe the digestive system.

Spice	Use
Chili Pepper Varieties	Works as a peripheral circulatory stimulant, antispasmodic, a stimulant (local and general), mucolytic, and rubefacient (topically). It can be used in cases of spasms, cramps, sore muscles, poor circulation, and for those with a "cold" constitution, meaning they have a greater tendency to feel cold.
Cinnamon	It is astringent, mucilaginous, and antibacterial.
Cloves	Considered to be analgesic (pain-relieving), antibacterial, and antispasmodic. It is often used for toothache.
Cocoa/Cacao	An antioxidant and a stimulant.
Coriander	Can be used as a carminative.
Cumin	Antioxidant-rich and suitable for sootheing the digestive system.
Curry Leaf	Has been used as an antihelminthic (expels parasitic worms), tonic, stomachic (assists in digestions), carminative, analgesic, to reduce dysentery, to stop vomiting, and to reduce heat, thirst inflammation, and itching.
Dill Seed	An antispasmodic used to soothe the digestive system.
Fennel	A carminative that also has anti-inflammatory, aromatic, antimicrobial, and diuretic properties. Good for reducing flatulence.
Fenugreek	A galactagogue (helps nursing mothers with breast milk production) and an expectorant. It helps regulate blood sugar, cure constipation because of its mucilage content, and reduce digestive upset.
Galangal	Can be used to soothe digestion as a carminative.
Garlic	Is antibacterial, antiseptic, a circulatory stimulant, diaphoretic, diuretic, and antimicrobial. It can be used for high cholesterol, high blood pressure, common colds, and the flu.

Spice	Use
Ginger	Can be used as an anti-inflammatory, stimulant, diaphoretic, anodyne (reduces pain in the gastro-intestinal tract and warms and stimulates the stomach), and as a rubefacient (increase blood circulation on skin). It is best for poor peripheral circulation and poor appetite, dysmenorrhoea (period pain), extreme exhaustion, flatulence and nausea, acute colds, rheumatism, and arthritic conditions.
Green Cardamom	Used to soothe the digestive system.
Green Tea	Can be stimulating or calming, due to its caffeine and theanine content, respectively. It is also nootropic and antioxidant-rich.
Hibiscus and Roselle	Both are thought to be a source of antioxidants, such as anthocyanins, and may act as blood-pressure and cholesterol-modulating agents.
Horseradish	Is a mucolytic, a circulatory stimulant, and can be used in sinusitis and mucus congestion.
Juniper Berries	Are antiseptic, stimulant, carminative, and a general diuretic.
Licorice	Is anti-inflammatory, mucilaginous, antiviral, and anti-androgenic. It can be used for sore throats, colds and flus, nervous exhaustion, stress, fatigue, androgen-related acne, to soothe the stomach and gastrointestinal lining, and to aid *H. pylori* eradication.
Mustard	Can act as a counter-stimulant on the skin and a warming circulating stimulant in the body.
Myrrh	Is anti-inflammatory, wound healing, astringent, and antiseptic. It is helpful for treating sore, dry throats, sore mouths, and ulcers, and is great for improving skin conditions.
Nigella Seed	Is an immune modulator, anti-inflammatory, a digestive aid, and has antiseptic properties. It is also helpful for weight loss, low immune system function, and poor digestion.

Spice	Use
Nutmeg	Thought to be antiemetic, carminative, spasmolytic, orexigenic (appetite stimulant), a gastric secretion stimulant, an inhibitor of prostaglandin, and an aphrodisiac.
Onion	Has been known to be a mucolytic, anti-inflammatory, and antibacterial, and has been used for the common cold, influenza, for sore throats, and for general immune system health.
Peppermint	Is antibacterial, antispasmodic, carminative, stomachic, a stimulant, a local anesthetic, and it is cooling because of menthol. Peppermint is good for the common cold, the digestive system, influenza, managing fevers, reducing inflammation in the throat, relieving toothaches, and as a cooling mouthwash.
Rose	Is calming, a mild nervine, astringent and antibacterial, bactericidal, antidepressant, a heart tonic, a stomachic, and a depurative.
Rosemary	Is an antioxidant and can aid liver detoxification. It is hepatoproctive (liver protecting), a nervine, a relaxing tonic, a peripheral circulatory stimulator, an astringent, and a diuretic. It is indicated in certain liver conditions, can help improve memory, reduce stress, and is a nootropic.
Saffron	Is potentially antiedematogenic and potentially antinociceptive (stops pain). It is thought to have anti-inflammatory properties and is used to treat depression.
Sage	Is an antihyperhidrotic, antibacterial, astringent, stimulant, and carminative. It can be used for sore, dry throats, inflammation in the mouth and throat, menopausal hot flashes, to reduce excess sweating and perspiration, inflammation of the skin, flatulence, poor digestion, and mild dyspepsia.
Star Anise	Has antimicrobial properties and has traditionally been used as a carminative.

Spice	Use
Sumac	Has been shown to have antibacterial, hepatoprotective, antifungal, antioxidant, anti-inflammatory, DNA protective, anti-ischemic, and vasorelaxant activities, among other actions.
Szechuan Pepper	Stimulates saliva and can numb the mouth.
Thyme	Has antibacterial properties and is indicated for use in colds, the flu, sore throats, and coughs.
Turmeric	Is anti-inflammatory, antioxidant, and antibacterial, and it is thought to have effects on Alzheimer's.
Vanilla	Often thought to be an aphrodisiac.
Wild Celery Seed	Can be used as a diuretic, anti-inflammatory, and pain-reliever (as a secondary action).

Standard U.S./Metric Measurement Conversions

VOLUME CONVERSIONS	
U.S. Volume Measure	**Metric Equivalent**
⅛ teaspoon	0.5 milliliter
¼ teaspoon	1 milliliter
½ teaspoon	2 milliliters
1 teaspoon	5 milliliters
½ tablespoon	7 milliliters
1 tablespoon (3 teaspoons)	15 milliliters
2 tablespoons (1 fluid ounce)	30 milliliters
¼ cup (4 tablespoons)	60 milliliters
⅓ cup	90 milliliters
½ cup (4 fluid ounces)	125 milliliters
⅔ cup	160 milliliters
¾ cup (6 fluid ounces)	180 milliliters
1 cup (16 tablespoons)	250 milliliters
1 pint (2 cups)	500 milliliters
1 quart (4 cups)	1 liter (about)

WEIGHT CONVERSIONS	
U.S. Weight Measure	**Metric Equivalent**
½ ounce	15 grams
1 ounce	30 grams
2 ounces	60 grams
3 ounces	85 grams
¼ pound (4 ounces)	115 grams
½ pound (8 ounces)	225 grams
¾ pound (12 ounces)	340 grams
1 pound (16 ounces)	454 grams

OVEN TEMPERATURE CONVERSIONS

Degrees Fahrenheit	Degrees Celsius
200 degrees F	95 degrees C
250 degrees F	120 degrees C
275 degrees F	135 degrees C
300 degrees F	150 degrees C
325 degrees F	160 degrees C
350 degrees F	180 degrees C
375 degrees F	190 degrees C
400 degrees F	205 degrees C
425 degrees F	220 degrees C
450 degrees F	230 degrees C

BAKING PAN SIZES

American	Metric
8 x 1½ inch round baking pan	20 x 4 cm cake tin
9 x 1½ inch round baking pan	23 x 3.5 cm cake tin
11 x 7 x 1½ inch baking pan	28 x 18 x 4 cm baking tin
13 x 9 x 2 inch baking pan	30 x 20 x 5 cm baking tin
2 quart rectangular baking dish	30 x 20 x 3 cm baking tin
15 x 10 x 2 inch baking pan	30 x 25 x 2 cm baking tin (Swiss roll tin)
9 inch pie plate	22 x 4 or 23 x 4 cm pie plate
7 or 8 inch springform pan	18 or 20 cm springform or loose bottom cake tin
9 x 5 x 3 inch loaf pan	23 x 13 x 7 cm or 2 lb narrow loaf or pate tin
1½ quart casserole	1.5 liter casserole
2 quart casserole	2 liter casserole

Index